Physiology of Sport and Exercise

Physiology of
Sport and Exercise

Jeremy Browning

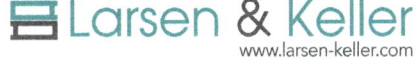

www.larsen-keller.com

Physiology of Sport and Exercise
Jeremy Browning
ISBN: 978-1-64172-508-8 (Hardback)

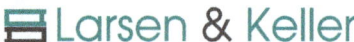 Larsen & Keller

Published by Larsen and Keller Education,
5 Penn Plaza,
19th Floor,
New York, NY 10001, USA

Cataloging-in-Publication Data

Physiology of sport and exercise / Jeremy Browning.
    p. cm.
Includes bibliographical references and index.
ISBN 978-1-64172-508-8
1. Exercise--Physiological aspects. 2. Sports--Physiological aspects.
3. Physical fitness--Physiological aspects. I. Browning, Jeremy.
QP301 .P49 2020
612.044--dc23

For more information regarding Larsen and Keller Education and its products, please visit the publisher's website www.larsen-keller.com

Table of Contents

Preface

This book is a culmination of my many years of practice in this field. I attribute the success of this book to my support group. I would like to thank my parents who have showered me with unconditional love and support and my peers and professors for their constant guidance.

The physiology of physical exercise is known as exercise physiology. It includes the study of acute responses and chronic adaptations to exercise. It closely observes and examines the effects of exercise including changes in cardiovascular, muscular, and neurohumoral systems. It also leads to changes in the strength and functional capacity due to endurance training. The effect of training on the body is the reaction to the adaptive responses of the body that arise from exercise. This field is also involved in studying the effect of exercise on pathology along with the mechanisms by which exercise can reduce or reverse disease progression. This book is a compilation of chapters that discuss the most vital concepts in the field of exercise physiology. It aims to shed light on some of the unexplored aspects of this field. The book is appropriate for those seeking detailed information in this area.

The details of chapters are provided below for a progressive learning:

Chapter – What is Exercise Physiology?

Exercise physiology deals with the study of physiology of physical exercise. It studies the responses and chronic adaptations to exercise. The topics elaborated in this chapter will help in gaining a better perspective about exercise, exercise physiology, adaptations to exercise and sports physiology.

Chapter – Optimal Nutrition for Exercise

Optimal nutrition is necessary to supply the nutrient for tissue maintenance, repair and growth. Energy and nutrients mainly come from three macronutrients, namely, carbohydrates, proteins and fats. This chapter closely examines these macronutrients to provide an extensive understanding of the subject.

Chapter – Aerobic Exercise

Aerobic exercise is a form of physical exercise which depends on the aerobic energy generating process for a low to high intensity workout. Some of its types are water aerobics, endurance training, cross training, etc. This chapter has been carefully written to provide an easy understanding of these components of aerobic exercise.

Chapter – Anaerobic Exercise

A type of physical exercise which is used by athletes in non-endurance sports for improvement in strength, speed and power is referred to as anaerobic exercise. A few of such exercises are strength training, stretching and sprinting. This chapter has been carefully written to provide an easy understanding of these anaerobic exercises.

Chapter – Effects of Exercise

There are many effects of exercise which can be categorized into positive and negative effects. Some of its positive effects are improvement in agility, flexibility and physical fitness. A few of its negative effects include muscle soreness, hyponatremia, muscle cramps, etc. This chapter discusses in detail these positive and negative effects of exercise.

Chapter – Diverse Aspects of Exercise Physiology

The diverse aspects of exercise physiology can be classified as lactace threshold, physical literacy, strength training, exercise intolerance, metabolic equivalent of task (MET), etc. The topics elaborated in this chapter will help in gaining a better perspective about these aspects of exercise physiology.

Jeremy Browning

1

What is Exercise Physiology?

Exercise physiology deals with the study of physiology of physical exercise. It studies the responses and chronic adaptations to exercise. The topics elaborated in this chapter will help in gaining a better perspective about exercise, exercise physiology, adaptations to exercise and sports physiology.

Exercise

Exercise is the training of the body to improve its function and enhance its fitness.

The terms exercise and physical activity are often used interchangeably, Physical activity is an inclusive term that refers to any expenditure of energy brought about by bodily movement via the skeletal muscles; as such, it includes the complete spectrum of activity from very low resting levels to maximal exertion. Exercise is a component of physical activity. The distinguishing characteristic of exercise is that it is a structured activity specifically planned to develop and maintain physical fitness. Physical conditioning refers to the development of physical fitness through the adaptation of the body and its various systems to an exercise program.

Types of Physical Fitness

Physical fitness is a general concept and is defined in many ways by different scientists. Physical fitness is discussed here in two major categories: health-related physical fitness and motor-performance physical fitness. Despite some overlap between these classifications, there are major differences, as described below.

Health-related Physical Fitness

Health-related physical fitness is defined as fitness related to some aspect of health. This type of physical fitness is primarily influenced by an individual's exercise habits; thus, it is a dynamic state and may change. Physical characteristics that constitute health-related physical fitness include strength and endurance of skeletal muscles, joint flexibility, body composition, and cardiorespiratory endurance. All these attributes change in response to appropriate physical conditioning programs, and all are related to health.

Strength and endurance of skeletal muscles of the trunk help maintain correct posture and prevent such problems as low back pain. Minimal levels of muscular strength and endurance are needed for routine tasks of living, such as carrying bags of groceries or picking up a young child. Individuals with very low levels of muscular strength and endurance are limited in the performance of routine tasks and have to lead a restricted life. Such limitations are perhaps only indirectly related to health, but individuals who cannot pick up and hug a grandchild or must struggle to get up from a soft chair surely have a lower quality of life than that enjoyed by their fitter peers.

Flexibility, or range of motion around the joints, also ranks as an important component of health-related fitness. Lack of flexibility in the lower back and posterior thigh is thought to contribute to low back pain. Extreme lack of flexibility also has a deleterious effect on the quality of life by limiting performance.

Body composition refers to the ratio between fat and lean tissue in the body. Excess body fat is clearly related to several health problems, including cardiovascular disease, type 2 (adult-onset) diabetes mellitus, and certain forms of cancer. Body composition is affected by diet, but exercise habits play a crucial role in preventing obesity and maintaining acceptable levels of body fat.

Cardiorespiratory endurance, or aerobic fitness, is probably what most people identify as physical fitness. Aerobic fitness refers to the integrated functional capacity of the heart, lungs, vascular system, and skeletal muscles to expend energy. The basic activity that underlies this type of fitness is aerobic metabolism in the muscle cell, a process in which oxygen is combined with a fuel source (fats or carbohydrates) to release energy and produce carbon dioxide and water. The energy is used by the muscle to contract, thereby exerting force that can be used for movement. For the aerobic reaction to take place, the cardiorespiratory system (i.e., the circulatory and pulmonary systems) must constantly supply oxygen and fuel to the muscle cell and remove carbon dioxide from it. The maximal rate at which aerobic metabolism can occur is thus determined by the functional capacity of the cardiorespiratory system and is measured in the laboratory as maximal oxygen intake. As will be discussed in detail below, aerobic fitness is inversely related to the incidence of coronary heart disease and hypertension.

Motor-performance Physical Fitness

Motor-performance fitness is defined as the ability of the neuromuscular system to perform specific tasks. Test items used to assess motor-performance fitness include chin-ups, sit-ups, the 50-yard dash, the standing long jump, and the shuttle run (a timed run in which the participant dashes back and forth between two points). The primary physical characteristics measured by these tests are the strength and endurance of the skeletal muscles and the speed or power of the legs. These traits are important for success in many types of athletics.

There is disagreement among experts about the relative importance of health-related and motor-performance physical fitness. While both types of fitness are obviously desirable, their relative values should be determined by an individual's personal fitness objectives. If success in athletic events is of primary importance, motor-performance fitness should be emphasized. If concern about health is paramount, health-related fitness should be the focus. Different types of fitness may be important not only to different individuals but also to the same individual at different times. The 16-year-old competing on a school athletic team is likely to focus on motor performance. The typical middle-aged individual is not as likely to be concerned about athletic success, emphasizing instead health and appearance. One further point should be made: to a great extent, motor-performance physical fitness is determined by genetic potential. The person who can run fast at 10 years of age will be fast at age 17; although training may enhance racing performance, it will not appreciably change the individual's genetically determined running speed. On the other hand, characteristics of health-related physical fitness, while also partly determined by inheritance, are much more profoundly influenced by exercise habits.

Principles of Exercise Training

Research in exercise training has led to the recognition of a number of general principles of conditioning. These principles must be applied to the development of a successful exercise program.

Specificity

The principle of specificity derives from the observation that the adaptation of the body or change in physical fitness is specific to the type of training undertaken. Quite simply this means that if a fitness objective is to increase flexibility, then flexibility training must be used. If one desires to develop strength, resistance or strengthening exercises must be employed. This principle is indeed simple; however, it is frequently ignored. Many fraudulent claims for an exercise product or system promise overall physical fitness from one simple training technique. A person should be suspicious of such claims and should consider whether or not the exercise training recommended is the type that will produce the specific changes desired.

Overload

Overload, the second important principle, means that to improve any aspect of physical fitness the individual must continually increase the demands placed on the appropriate body systems. For example, to develop strength, progressively heavier objects must be lifted. Overload in running programs is achieved by running longer distances or by increasing the speed.

Progression

Individuals frequently make the mistake of attempting too rapid a fitness change. A classic example is that of the middle-aged man or woman who has done no exercise for 20 years and suddenly begins a vigorous training program. The result of such activity is frequently an injury or, at the least, stiffness and soreness. There are no hard-and-fast rules on how rapidly one should progress to a higher level of activity. The individual's subjective impression of whether or not the body seems to be able to tolerate increased training serves as a good guide. In general it might be reasonable not to progress to higher levels of activity more often than every one or two weeks.

Warm-up/Cool Down

Another important practice to follow in an exercise program is to gradually start the exercise session and gradually taper off at the end. The warm-up allows various body systems to adjust to increased metabolic demands. The heart rate increases, blood flow increases, and muscle temperatures rise.

Warming up is certainly a more comfortable way to begin an exercise session and is probably safer. Progressively more vigorous exercises or a gradual increase in walking speed are good ways to warm up. It is equally important to cool down—that is, to gradually reduce exercise intensity—at the end of each session. The abrupt cessation of vigorous exercise may cause blood to pool in the legs, which can cause fainting or, more seriously, can sometimes precipitate cardiac complications. Slow walking and stretching for five minutes at the end of an exercise session is therefore a good practice. The heart rate should gradually decline during the cool down, and by the end of the five minutes it should be less than 120 beats per minute for individuals under 50 years of age and less than 100 beats per minute for those over 50.

Frequency, Intensity and Duration

To provide guidance on how much exercise an individual should do, exercise physiologists have developed equations based on research. It is generally agreed that to develop and maintain physical fitness, the exercise must be performed on a regular basis. A frequency of about every other day or three days per week appears minimally sufficient. Many individuals exercise more frequently than this, and, of course, such additional exercise is acceptable provided that one does not become overtrained and suffer illness or injury.

The intensity of exercise required to produce benefits has been the subject of much study. Many people have the impression that exercise is not doing any good unless it hurts. This is simply not true. Regular exercise at 45 to 50 percent of one's maximal capacity is adequate to improve one's physiological functioning and overall health. This level of intensity is generally comfortable for most individuals. A reliable way to gauge exercise intensity is to measure the heart rate during exercise. An exercise heart rate that is 65 percent of a person's maximal heart rate corresponds to approximately 50 percent of his maximal capacity. Maximal heart rate can be estimated by subtracting one's age in years from 220 (or, in the case of active males, by subtracting half of one's age from 205). Thus, a sedentary 40-year-old man has an estimated maximal heart rate of 180 beats per minute. Sixty-five percent of this maximal rate is 117 beats per minute; thus by exercising at 117 beats per minute, this individual is working at about 50 percent of his maximal capacity. To determine exercising heart rate, a person should exercise for several minutes, to allow the heart rate to adjust. The exerciser should then stop exercising, quickly find the pulse, and count the number of beats for 15 seconds. Multiplying this by four gives the rate in beats per minute. The pulse must be taken immediately after stopping exercise, since the heart rate rapidly begins to return to the resting level after work has been stopped. As noted above, exercising at the 50 percent level of intensity will improve physiologic functioning and provide health benefits. This level of exercise will not produce the maximum fitness needed for competitive athletics.

Overall Conditioning

Much emphasis has been given in the foregoing discussion to aerobic fitness, because this form of conditioning is extremely important. It should be noted, however, that other types of conditioning also have benefits. A total exercise program should include strengthening exercises, to maintain body mass and appropriate levels of strength for daily functioning, and stretching exercises to maintain joint mobility and flexibility. The specificity principle described above indicates that no one exercise is likely to produce the overall conditioning effect. In general, an exercise plan should consist of aerobics, exercises that increase the strength and endurance of various skeletal muscle groups, and flexibility exercises to maintain good joint function.

Individual Differences

The principles of exercise training should be viewed as general guidelines. Individuals differ in both physiological and psychological adaptations to exercise. Two people who are similar in many respects and who start the same exercise program may have entirely different impressions of it. One person may feel that the exercise is too easy, while the other may believe that it is much too hard. It is certainly appropriate that the exercise plan be adjusted to account for preferences. Likewise, some individuals will progress to more intense training levels far more rapidly than others do. As mentioned earlier, exercise progress should be adjusted according to the exerciser's own assessment.

Individuals also differ in the type of exercise they like or can tolerate. Jogging, for instance, is not for everyone. Many people who dislike jogging, or who suffer running injuries, can find other satisfactory exercise activities, such as cycling, walking, swimming, or participating in a sport. Many kinds of exercise activities are appropriate and can provide physiological and health benefits to the participant. There is no one best exercise.

Risks of Exercise

Regular participation in an exercise program can provide several benefits. Yet exercise is similar to other medical or health interventions in that there are also potential costs associated with the activity. These costs range from minor inconveniences, such as time taken up by exercise, to more serious complications, including injury and even sudden death.

Injuries

It is clear that some people who participate in exercise training will develop injuries to their bones, muscles, and joints. Despite unfounded reports in the mass media of extremely high injury rates among adult exercisers, there have been few good studies of exercise injuries in populations. One of the difficulties in performing such studies has been the need to identify both the number of cases (individuals who become injured) and the number of persons at risk for injury (the total number of individuals exercising in the population). These two figures are necessary in order to calculate true injury rates. The best available studies on injury rates suggest that about 25 to 30 percent of adult runners will become injured over the course of a year, if injury is defined as an incident that causes an individual to stop exercising for at least one week. If only more serious injuries, such as those for which the individual seeks medical care, are considered, injury rates are much lower, perhaps in the range of 1 percent per year.

Little is known about the causes of exercise injuries. One factor that has been linked to injury is the amount of exercise; for example, individuals who run more miles are likelier to be injured than those who run fewer miles. Factors such as age, sex, body type, and experience have not been shown to be associated with risk of injury. It seems logical that structural abnormalities, sudden increases in training intensity, and types of equipment used are likely to be related to injury risk; however, data to support these opinions are not available.

In view of the limited scientific data on injury risk, the exerciser is advised to follow common-sense practices until such time as the causes of injury are better understood. Exercisers should start their program slowly and gradually progress to more intensive training levels. They should use good equipment and pay particular attention to proper footwear. Exercisers who have had previous injuries should recognize that they may be more susceptible to similar injuries in the future. All exercisers should use caution and should monitor their bodies for the early warning signs of injury. If a problem begins to develop, it is good advice to stop exercising or to reduce the intensity of training for a few days to see if the problem disappears. Exercisers should not be afraid to experiment on themselves to find out what training practices and techniques seem to be more comfortable and less likely to produce injury. Moderation is good advice, few injuries are reported in individuals who run 10 to 15 miles per week, and this level is adequate to provide many health benefits.

Sudden Death

Obviously, the most serious complication from an exercise program is sudden death. This is, fortunately, a rare occurrence. As discussed earlier, several studies have shown that individuals who regularly participate in exercise have a lower risk of dying from a heart attack. There is, however, also evidence that suggests a higher risk of dying during exercise than during sedentary activities. When one considers the total risk of sudden death over a 24-hour period, regular exercisers are much less likely to experience this catastrophe.

Virtually all individuals who drop dead suddenly have advanced coronary heart disease. It follows, therefore, that the best way to reduce the risk of sudden death during exercise is to avoid getting advanced coronary heart disease. This implies following good health practices in other aspects of life, such as not smoking, eating a prudent diet, and maintaining an ideal body weight. Individuals who are middle-aged or older can probably reduce their risk of sudden death by knowing about their coronary risk status and their general state of health before undertaking an exercise program. There are, of course, no guarantees, but if an individual has a thorough examination by a competent physician, including a maximal exercise test and other procedures that screen for coronary heart disease, that person can probably safely begin an exercise program.

Agility Exercises for Athletes

Agility is defined as an athlete's ability to move at an accelerated pace in one direction and then instantly decelerate and shift position within a matter of seconds. It is the one facet of sports training that can separate a good athlete from a great one.

Whatever sports you engage in, these agility drills can improve your performance by strengthening the joints and muscles that go largely untested in daily life. As with any type of sports training, start slowly and focus on maintaining proper form. This will not only help you develop the stability needed to perform at your best, it can significantly reduce your risk of injury.

Plyometric Agility Hurdles

Athletes often use plyometric jumping exercises to build power and improve coordination. Hurdles are not only vital to training for field sports, they can improve the strength and jumping ability of basketball players, skiers, figure skaters, and sports divers. This exercise should only be performed after a thorough warm-up.

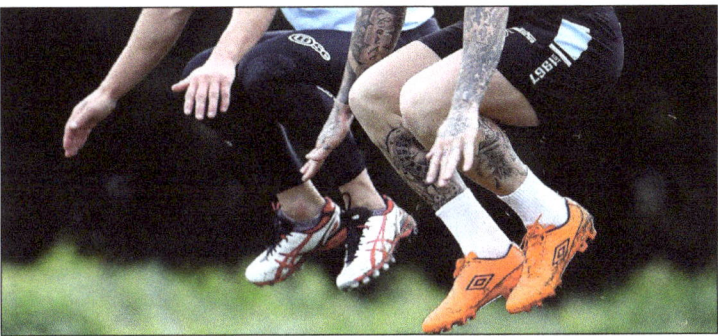

To do plyometric agility hurdles:

- Set up a series of low agility hurdles in two-foot increments.

- Starting with legs shoulder-width apart, jump upward and forward to clear each hurdle, landing on the balls of your feet.

- Upon landing, jump again, driving forward with your arms.

- Repeat for 10 to 12 repetitions ("reps") for one set. Rest for about a minute and complete two more sets.

You can perform the same drill with only the right foot and then only the left foot. As you improve, move the hurdles further apart.

Speed Ladder Agility Drills

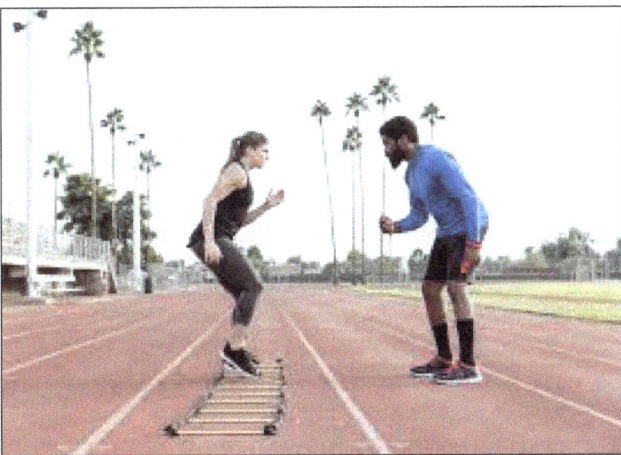

The speed ladder is a simple piece of portable equipment that can be used to perform the following agility drills:

- The forward-running, high-knee drill is great for improving foot speed and coordination. Run with high knees through the ladder, touching every ladder space. Land on the balls of the feet and drive forward with your arms. Repeat for a total of three sets.

- The lateral-running, side-to-side drill is ideal for court-sports, improving both knee and ankle stability. Keeping a low center of gravity, step side-to-side through the ladder one foot at a time. Touch in each rung of the ladder with both feet. Land on the balls of the feet. Repeat right to left and left to right for a total of three sets.

Plyometric Box Drills

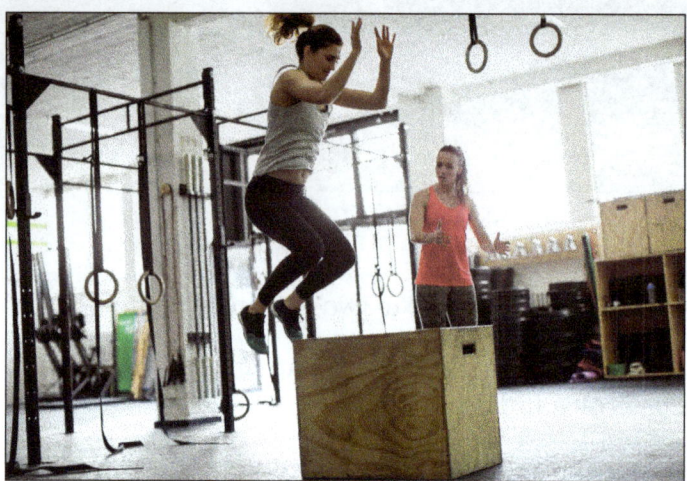

Plyometric box drills are a great way to build explosive power and foot speed. A plyometric box is a padded or unpadded cube that is anywhere from 14 to 36 inches in height.

Among some of the more popular plyo box drills:

- For step-ups, start by standing in front of the box. Step up onto the box with one leg, then bring the other leg up as you straighten both legs. Step back down and repeat on the opposite side for one rep. Repeat 10 times for one set. Complete three sets.

- For lateral stepovers, start by standing to the side of the box. Step laterally onto the box with one leg, then bring the other leg up so that you're standing on top of the box. Step down with one leg, then bring the other leg down to the ground. Continue for one set of 10 reps. Complete three sets.

- For box jumps, start by standing in front of the box. Jump up onto the box, landing with both feet. Jump back down from the box, then immediately jump back up. Continue of one set of 10 reps. Complete three sets.

Lateral Plyometric Jumps

Lateral plyometric jumps help build dynamic power, coordination, and balance by using just an athlete's body weight. This advanced exercise is a must for any athlete who needs lateral power and coordination. Start slowly and gradually increase the height of the barrier.

To do a lateral plyometric jump:

- Lay a string or length of masking tape on a carpeted floor, lawn, or gym floor. Avoid doing this drill on a concrete floor.

- Standing on one side of the line with your feet no more than a hip-width apart, bend your knees to a deep squat position.

- Pushing through your heels, propel yourself upward and sideways to the other side of the line. Land softly and absorb the shock by squatting deeply.

- Repeat jumping back and forth over the line, keeping your shoulders and hips square and facing forward. Continue for 30 to 60 seconds for one set.

- Rest and complete two more sets.

As you get stronger, you can jump over exercise steps and even low hurdles.

Tuck Jumps

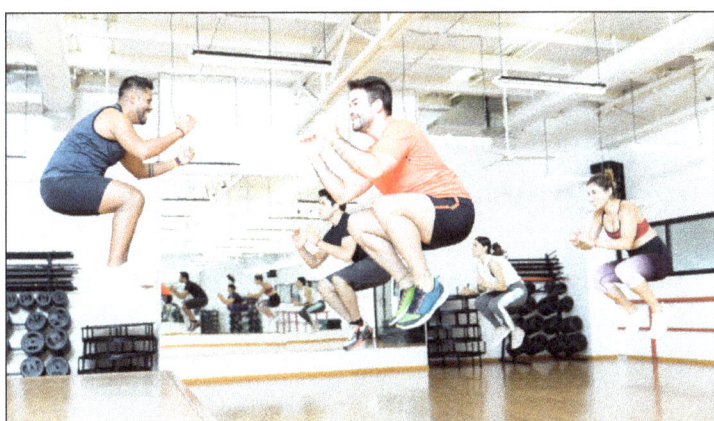

Tuck jumps are simple drills that improve your agility and power without the need for equipment. They not only strengthen the quadriceps muscles, they fully engage the core and hip flexors that lift your knee toward your body.

To do a standard tuck jump:

- Stand with your feet shoulder-width apart with your knees slightly bent.

- Bend your knees and jump straight up, bringing your knees to your chest while in midair.

- Grasp your knees quickly with your arms and let go.

- Upon landing, immediately repeat the next jump for a total of 10 to 12 reps. Rest and complete two more sets.

Dot Drills

Dot drills develop dynamic leg strength while increasing knee and ankle strength and stability. This is a great drill for any sport that requires quick changes of direction and solid landings (including soccer, basketball, racquetball, and skiing).

To do the dot drill, you will either need to purchase a dot drill mat or place five tape marks on the ground in the same pattern as the five dice.

The dot drill involves three exercises:

- For exercise one, start with your feet on two dots on one side of the square. Jump to the center dot with both feet, and then jump to the two dots on the opposite end of the square. Jumping backward to the center dot and back to the starting position for one rep. Continue for a total of six reps per set. Complete three sets.

- For exercise two, follow the same pattern as exercise one, but instead of jumping backward, jump up and spin around 180 degrees before continuing back the starting position. Complete three sets of six reps.

- For exercise three, start with your feet on two dots on one side of the square. Following one step after the next, move your right foot the center dot, left foot to the forward dot, right foot to the forward dot, left foot the center dot, right foot back to the starting dot, and left foot back to the starting dot. Continue, picking up speed, for a total of six reps. Complete three sets.

Exercise Physiology

Exercise physiology is the study of the body's responses to physical activity. These responses include changes in metabolism and in physiology of different areas of the body like the heart, lungs, and muscles, and structural changes in cells.

Exercise has been regarded as important to human health for thousands of years, beginning with ancient cultures. The Greek physician Hippocrates is one of the earliest-recorded and most well-known proponents of exercise. He recommended moderate exercise in order to stay healthy and even improve health. Other prominent ancient scholars throughout history followed suit, including Plato, Aristotle, and the Roman physician Galen, who believed that exercise improved general health, metabolism, and muscle tone, and even led to better bowel movements. Later, the Persian physician Avicenna also wrote in support of Galen in the medical text *Canon of Medicine*. Avicenna believed that exercise balanced the four body humors (an idea that was popular at the time and had been passed down from Ancient Greece). Importantly, he also recognized that too much exercise could have negative effects on the body.

In the 16th Century, around the start of Scientific Revolution, physicians began to write books on exercise. One of the earliest known books on exercise was *Book of Bodily Exercise*, written by the Spanish physician Cristobal Mendez. In his book, Mendez discussed benefits, types, and values of exercise, along with common exercises and why they were important to perform. In the 19th Century, some medical textbooks began to include chapters on exercise. The negative effects of lack of exercise, including poor circulation, weakness, and increased likelihood of disease, became more well-known. As the importance of physical activity became more and more important, schools also began to offer physical education classes, which required students to perform exercises for a set period of time each day.

Laboratories devoted to the study of exercise physiology were also established in the 20th Century.

These included the Harvard Fatigue Laboratory, opened in 1927, and the Physical Fitness Research Laboratory at University of Illinois, opened in 1944. These schools conducted numerous on such topics as fatigue, cardiovascular changes during exercise, oxygen uptake by the body, and the effects of training. In 1948, the Journal of Applied Physiology began to be published. This journal publishes peer-reviewed research in exercise physiology and still exists today. While contributing greatly to our understanding of exercise's effects, exercise physiology labs also trained numerous scientists who would go on to found their own exercise physiology laboratories in universities and medical schools all over the world.

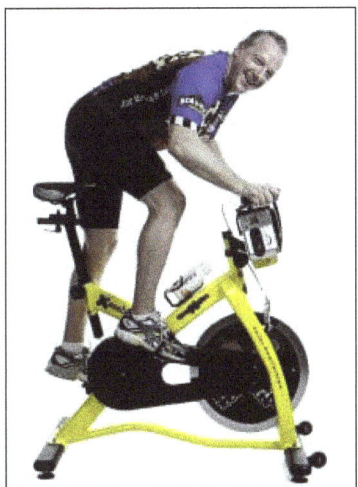

A variety of changes take place in the body during exercise.

Types of Exercise Physiology

The two types of exercise physiology are sport and clinical. Sport exercise physiology is, as its name suggests, related to athletes. Sport physiologists use knowledge of the body's response to exercise in order to develop training regimens for athletes. Such regimens include fitness conditioning, which is the process of training to become more physically fit through periods of exercising certain muscles and resting. Clinical exercise physiology is the use of physical activity for therapy, treatment, and prevention of chronic diseases. One disease that can be aided by exercise is diabetes. Exercise uses the body's stored glucose, so a diabetic may use exercise to help keep their blood sugar levels down. Another disease treated with exercise therapy is osteoporosis, the loss of bone tissue that commonly occurs in old age. Osteoporosis may cause joint pain and limit movement. Clinical exercise physiologists work with affected individuals to show them how to exercise in a safe way that minimizes pain, and may recommend activities such as swimming that are easier on the joints. Exercise is also sometimes used as part of a treatment for anxiety and depression, either as a standalone condition or as a result of a physical disease, because it raises serotonin levels and reduces stress.

Exercise physiology is also sometimes regarded as being either non-clinical or clinical; "non-clinical" is very similar to sport physiology, but the scope is widened to include healthy non-athletes who are looking to lose weight and/or gain fitness.

The Basic Principles in Exercise Physiology

The body's responses to a single bout of exercise are regulated by the principle of homeostasis.

Homeostasis is defined as the ability of the body to maintain a stable internal environment for cells by closely regulating various critical variables such as pH or acid base balance, oxygen tension, blood glucose concentration and body temperature.

The overload, specificity, reversibility and individuality principles influence training adaptations in the body, for health as well as performance.

The application of an specific and appropriate stressor can sometimes be referred to as overloading the system. The overload principle states that habitually overloading a system causes it to respond and adapt. The overload principle can be quantified according to load (intensity and duration), repetition, rest and frequency. Load refers to the intensity of the exercise stressor i.e in strength training it can refer to the amount of resistance or in swimming it can refer to speed. The greater the load, the greater the fatigue and recovery time needed. Repetition implies the number of times that a load is applied. Rest refers to the time interval between repetitions and frequency refers to the number of training sessions per week.

The specificity principle states that only the system or body part repeatedly stressed will adapt to chronic overload. Therefore the overload principle will only apply to the system or body part used while exercising. Reversibility states that whereas training may enhance performance, inactivity will lead to a decrease in performance.

The individuality principle states that while the physiological responses to a particular stressor can be mostly predictable, the precise responses and adaptations will still differ among individuals.

Musculoskeletal System

Exercise is about movement, and the muscular system is primarily responsible for creating movement. Therefore, the responses and adaptations of the muscular system to exercise are important parts of exercise physiology. During exercise, many changes take place in skeletal muscle, such as changes in temperature, acidity, and ion concentrations. These changes affect muscle performance and may lead to fatigue. Indeed, the mechanisms of muscle fatigue is an important area of inquiry in exercise physiology. In addition, the adaptations of the muscular system to exercise lead to long-term changes in exercise capability.

Depending on the type of exercise, changes in enzyme concentrations, contractile protein content, and vascularisation affect the ability of the muscle to perform work. For example, endurance exercise increases concentrations of enzymes in skeletal muscle that are involved in the aerobic production of energy. In contrast, strength training is associated with increases in the size of the muscle due to increased synthesis of contractile proteins, with little change in anaerobic enzyme content. These types of adaptations are appropriate for a certain type of activity in that these adaptations will improve muscle performance in the types of activities that stimulated these adaptations.

If muscles are under loaded, it does not matter how much they are exercised, they will increase little in strength. On the other side, if they are trained with at least 50 percent of maximal force of contraction, they will develop strength rapidly even if the contractions are performed only a few times each day. Using this principle, experiments on muscle building have shown that six nearly maximal muscle contractions performed in three sets 3 days a week give approximately optimal increase in muscle strength, without producing chronic muscle fatigue.

The musculoskeletal system is fundamental in exercise physiology. The strength of a muscle is mostly determined by its cross sectional area. Therefore size is key.

Mechanical Work performed by a muscle is the amount of force applied by the muscle multiplied by the distance over which the force is applied.

Muscle Strength is the maximal amount of tension or force that a muscle or a muscle group can voluntarily exert on a maximal effort when the type of muscle contraction, segment velocity and joint angle is specified.

The power of muscle contraction is different from muscle strength because power is a measure of the total amount of work that the muscle performs in a unit period of time and is generally measured in kilogram meters (kg-m) per minute.

Another important concept is endurance, defined as the ability to perform repeated contractions against a resistance or maintain a contraction for a period of time.

Types of Skeletal Muscle Actions

There are several types of skeletal muscle actions:

- Static (Isometric): it occurs when tension is developed in the muscle without movement, therefore the muscle origin and insertion does not move and there is no changes in muscle length. During a static muscle contraction, the myosin and actin myofilaments form cross-bridges and generate force, but the external force is greater than the muscle-produced force. No mechanical work (force x distance) is done, as there is no displacement, even though there is energy expenditure.

- Dynamic (Isotonic) Muscle Actions:

  ○ Concentric: The muscle produces enough force to overcome the external resistance. The muscle shortens and there is movement at the joint. The myosin and actin myofilaments form cross-bridges, and the filaments slide past each other causing muscle shortening. Energy expenditure results in positive mechanical work as force production and displacement occurs.

  ○ Eccentric: The muscle lengthens while producing force. This happens because the external resistance moves in the direction opposite to the standard concentric (shortening) action. A high force is produced by the contractile elements and this makes these type of muscle actions an important training stimulus. Eccentric muscle actions are also associated with muscle damage and soreness and it is advised that the eccentric component of exercise training should initially be limited. Furthermore, eccentric contractions have clinical value during the rehabilitation of tendinopathies.

- Dynamic (Isokinetic) Muscle Actions: These muscle actions are characterised by constant velocity and can only be achieved in a laboratory or clinic setting. Specialised computerised equipment is necessary to maximise resistance at every angle of range of motion. The isokinetic contractions can be concentric or eccentric. These type of contractions and devices can help athletes perform exercises that simulates the actual speed and sport-specific activities.

Skeletal Muscle Fibre Types

Human skeletal muscle fibres vary in terms of their mechanical, physiological and biochemical characteristics. Generally, human skeletal muscles have three types of fibres: Type I, Type IIa and Type IIx.

Fast Twitch (FT) or Type II fibers have two primary subdivisions, Type IIa and Type IIx. Type IIa fibres have intermediate properties - they are fast contracting fibres but also have a oxidative metabolic profile. Both Type IIa and Type IIx show rapid contraction speed, high capacity for anaerobic ATP production through glycolysis and a larger diameter. Type IIx fibres are fatigable fibres.

Slow Twitch (ST) or type I fibers generate energy primarily through aerobic system. This type of fibre shows a relatively slow contraction speed, a higher number of larger mitochondria and larger amounts of myoglobin. These fibres are the slow, oxidative, fatigue-resistant fibres.

Muscle Hypertrophy

Muscle sizes are determined mainly by genetic and anabolic hormone secretion. Training can add another 30 to 60 percent of muscle hypertrophy, mostly from increased muscle fibers diameter, but in a small part also from increased number of fibers (hyperplasia).

Hypertrophied muscle are characterized by:

- An increased number of myofibrils;

- Increased number of mitochondrial enzymes;

- Increase in ATP and phosphocreatine amounts available;

- Increased stored glycogen and triglyceride;

- Thus enhancing both aerobic and anaerobic systems.

Muscle Strength Determinants

The amount of force that a muscle can generate varies individually. Genetics play a big role in this force generation, but there are other determinants as well:

- Nerve supply: The number of motor units recruited determine the amount of force. Slow twitch (Type I fibre) motor units are easily recruited, whereas Fast twitch (Type IIx) motor units hold more muscle fibres and can therefore generate more force.

- Muscle length: Most force is produced when muscles are working in mid-range. Mid-range is the position where there is optimal overlap of the thin and thick filaments at sarcomere level.

- Speed of shortening: More force is generated with slower movement. A dynamic (isotonic) muscle action produces more force than a static (isometric) contraction.

- Mechanical advantage: Most muscles work at a mechanical disadvantage due to the position of the muscle insertion point in relation to the portion of the limb being moved. (Think of knee extension, where the quadriceps acts across the bone levers of the femur and tibia, the knee joint is the fulcrum and the quadriceps inserting onto the upper end of the tibia).

- Muscle fibre pennation: The fascicles in muscle are arranged according to the shape of the muscle. More force will be produced by muscles where the fascicles are parallel with the longitudinal axis of the muscle.

- Connective tissue: Connective tissue in and around the muscle provides support and also increases the muscle's ability to produce force.

Energy Systems

With respect to exercise, the area of metabolism involves the study of how the body generates energy for muscular work. The energy for exercise, in the form of adenosine triphosphate (ATP), is derived from the breakdown of food from the diet. Originally in the form of protein, fat, and carbohydrate, the energy is made available by different enzymatic pathways that break down food and ultimately lead to ATP formation. The specific metabolic pathway used and the associated food broken down for energy are affected by the type of exercise and length of time that a person is performing and have implications for the ability of the person to perform that exercise. These are important issues in exercise physiology because they affect decisions regarding the type, intensity, and duration of exercise to be prescribed to an athlete.

In order to meet the increased demands for ATP when exercising, there is an increase in the chemical reactions in the body providing ATP. In aerobic metabolism, the chemical reactions use oxygen to completely break down carbohydrates e.g. glycogen, glucose and fats for energy. With moderate levels of exercise, the muscles can use aerobic metabolism to meet the increased energy requirements. Aerobic metabolism does not allow for maximum power output of the muscles but aerobic activity can be sustained for long periods of time. The body first uses the stored oxygen available in the body and then the exercise level is limited by the capacities of the respiratory and cardiovascular systems to provide more oxygen to the active cells.

These systems do not work on a on-off base but rather in a conveniently mixed mode with considerable overlap between them.

Phosphocreatine-Creatine System

Phosphocreatine is another chemical compound that has a high-energy phosphate bond that can be hydrolysed to provide energy and resynthesize ATP. This occurs within a small fraction of a second. Therefore, all the energy stored in the muscle phosphocreatine is almost instantaneously available for muscle contraction, just as is the energy stored in ATP.

At the start of exercise ATP is broken down into ADP + Pi, resulting in ATP being reformed by the creatine phosphate (CP) reaction. A phosphate is donated to ADP from CP to reform ATP. This method is the fastest and simplest way to produce energy for a muscle contraction. This energy source lasts for about 5 seconds as muscle cells only store a small amount of ATP and CP. This reaction provides energy for the start of the exercise and short-term high intensity exercise. This energy production is done without oxygen, thus an anaerobic method of energy production.

Thus, the energy from the phosphagen system (ATP and Phosphocreatine stored in the muscle) is used for maximal short bursts of muscle power.

Anaerobic Glycolysis (Lactic Acid System)

The stored glycogen in muscle can be split into glucose and the glucose then used for energy. Glycolysis is the first part of this process, which occurs without use of oxygen and, therefore, is said to be anaerobic metabolism. During glycolysis, each glucose molecule is split into two pyruvic acid molecules, and energy is released to form four ATP molecules for each original glucose molecule.

These pyruvic acid molecules can then be used by mitochondria in muscle cells, reacting with oxygen and providing more ATP molecules (oxidative stage), but if the exercise is too intense then it is likely the oxygen is insufficient for this second stage to occur, therefore pyruvic acid is converted into lactic acid. By doing so considerable amount of ATP are formed without oxygen, but also of lactic acid which will diffuse into interstitial fluid and bloodstream.

Another characteristic of the glycogen-lactic acid system is that it can form ATP molecules about 2.5 times as rapidly as can the oxidative mechanism of the mitochondria. Therefore, when large amounts of ATP are required for short to moderate periods of muscle contraction, this anaerobic glycolysis mechanism can be used as a rapid source of energy. It is, however, only about one half as rapid as the phosphagen system. Under optimal conditions, the glycogen-lactic acid system can provide 1.3 to 1.6 minutes of maximal muscle activity in addition to the 8 to 10 seconds provided by the phosphagen system, although at somewhat reduced muscle power.

Oxidative Phosphorylation (Aerobic System)

The aerobic system is the oxidation of glucose, fatty acids and amino acids. Combined with oxygen these compounds are able to release great amounts of energy used to provide ATP. This occurs in the mitochondria of the cell. Two metabolic pathways, the Krebs cycle and the electron transport chain, work together. These pathways remove hydrogen from from carbohydrates, fats and proteins so that the potential energy in the hydrogen can be implemented to produce ATP.

This system provides less ATP per minute than the phosphagen system and the lactic acid system, but can last as long as there are nutrients to provide substrates.

The aerobic system is thus useful for less powerful but longer-term aerobic exercise activities.

Cardiovascular System

The cardiovascular system is responsible for the transport of blood, and therefore oxygen and nutrients, to the tissues of the body. Similarly, the cardiovascular system facilitates removal of waste products such as carbon dioxide from the body. In addition, the cardiovascular system is centrally involved in the dissipation of heat, which is critical during prolonged exercise.

The primary components of the cardiovascular system are the heart, which pumps the blood, and the arteries and veins, which carry the blood to and from the tissues. Although all systems (i.e. pulmonary, respiratory, skeletal muscle and cardiovascular system) are involved in constructing an appropriate response to exercise training, the cardiovascular system can be seen as the central hub. Therefore, a large proportion of study and research in exercise physiology focuses on the responses and adaptations of the cardiovascular system to exercise.

Important beneficial effects of exercise on the cardiovascular system include a decrease in resting blood pressure (an important risk factor in cardiovascular disease) and a decrease in blood cholesterol levels (reducing the risk for developing atherosclerosis). Furthermore, exercise is an important component of the cardiac rehabilitation process following a cardiac event such as a heart attack.

Individuals with training in exercise physiology are playing important roles in the research and implementation of exercise programs for the prevention of cardiovascular disease and the rehabilitation of individuals with cardiovascular disease.

Exercises increase some components of the cardiovascular system, such as:

- Stroke volume (SV)

- Cardiac output

- Systolic blood pressure (BP)

- Mean arterial pressure

To meet the metabolic demands of skeletal muscle during exercise, 2 major adjustments to blood flow must occur. First, cardiac output from the heart must increase. Second, blood flow from inactive organs and tissues must be redistributed to active skeletal muscle. At rest, muscles receive approximately 20% of the total blood flow, but during exercise, the blood flow to muscles increases to 80-85%.

Generally, the longer the duration of exercise, the greater the role the cardiovascular system plays in metabolism and performance during the exercise bout. An example would be the 100-meter sprint (little or no cardiovascular involvement) versus a marathon (maximal cardiovascular involvement).

Heart Rate

During exercise heart rate (HR) increases. This happens alongside oxygen uptake during exercise in order to reach steady-state heart rate during constant workload, sub-maximal exercise. In incremental maximal exercise heart rate increases up to maximal heart rate (HR_{max}). Initially cardiac output during exercise increases as a result of an increase in stroke volume. With a further increase in exercise workload, further increases in cardiac output becomes dependent on heart rate. In healthy people maximal exercise is limited by maximal heart rate (HR_{max}). Maximal heart rate can be estimated using the equation of 220 - age. In trained athletes an increase in stroke volume is noticed. This therefore allows for a greater cardiac output in trained individuals for a given heart rate.

Blood Flow and Pressure

During exercise various factors in the exercising muscle cause vasodilation and opening of dormant capillaries. These factors are:

- Increase in temperature.

- Decrease in oxygenation.

- Decrease in metabolic products.

As a result an significant increase in blood flow to the muscle is observed.

To maintain a sufficient blood pressure, systemically vasoconstriction causes blood to move from the periphery to the central circulation. This kept balance between vasoconstriction vasodilation, ensures that there is little change in blood pressure during steady-state exercise. During incremental exercise, the large increase in cardiac output required during high levels of exercise, can cause an increase in the systolic pressure up to around 200mmHg, but the diastolic pressure remains stable.

Pulmonary System

The pulmonary system is important for the exchange of oxygen and carbon dioxide between the air and blood. The primary component of the pulmonary system is the lungs, which vary in volume from 4-6L and if laid out flat would cover a huge surface area from 60 - 80m^2. Exercise places a great deal of stress on the pulmonary system as oxygen consumption and carbon dioxide production are increased during exercise, thus increasing the pulmonary ventilation rate. The control and regulation of the pulmonary system during exercise are areas of much research. As with the cardiovascular system, the interplay of exercise and the neurological control of breathing is not completely understood. Surprisingly, most evidence indicates that there are few, if any, adaptations to exercise in the pulmonary system itself in healthy individuals. However, adaptations in the musculature structures that controls breathing are apparent.

Oxygen Uptake.

Oxygen uptake (VO_2) is the amount of oxygen that the body takes up and utilises. Oxygen consumption rises exponentially during the first minutes of exercise, reaching a steady rate around the third minute and then remaining relatively stable. In such conditions, energy required by the working muscles and ATP production in aerobic metabolism are balanced, without lactate accumulation in blood.

VO_{2max} or Maximal Oxygen Uptake

Maximal oxygen consumption (VO_{2max}) is the region where oxygen consumption reach a steady state or increases only slightly with additional increases in exercise intensity. It provides a quantitative measures of a person's capacity for aerobic ATP resynthesis. Maximal oxygen uptake is dependent on a person's:

- Gender

- Height

- Weight

- Lung function

- Fitness level

- Type of activity being performed

VO_{2max} is exercise specific and is greater in activities involving large muscle groups. Trained athletes can have a higher Maximal Oxygen Uptake than sedentary individuals because of their enhanced stroke volume, improved myocardial function and a higher capacity for oxidative metabolism in active muscles. VO_{2max} in short-term studies is found to increase only 10% with the effect of training. However, that of a person who runs in marathons is 45% greater than that of an untrained person. This is believed to be partly genetically determined (e.g, stronger respiratory muscles, larger chest size in relation to body size) and partly due to long-term training.

Oxygen Diffusing Capacity

Oxygen diffusing capacity is a measure of the rate at which oxygen can diffuse from the alveoli into the blood. An increase in diffusing capacity is observed in a state of maximal exercise.

During exercise, increased blood flow through the lungs causes all of the pulmonary capillaries to be perfused at their maximal level, providing a greater surface area through which oxygen can diffuse into the pulmonary capillary blood. Athletes who require greater amounts of oxygen per minute have been found to have higher diffusing capacities.

Both arterial blood oxygen pressure and carbon dioxide pressure remains almost at normal level even during strenuous exercise, as they are well compensated.

Ventilation

During light to moderate intensity exercise/sports activities, ventilation increases linearly with oxygen uptake and carbon dioxide production. This is necessary to meet the body's oxygen requirement and to expel the additional produced carbon dioxide. Initially the increase in ventilation is achieved by an increase in the tidal volume, and with increasing demand by increasing the respiratory rate. During heavy to maximal exercise a rise in ventilation is observed in response to the lactate threshold. This is known as the ventilatory threshold. Should a person continue exercising a further rise in ventilation is observed at the onset of blood lactate accumulation (OBLA). This happens in order to expel more carbon dioxide in an effort to reduce the acidity in the blood. This rise in ventilation at the OBLA is known as respiratory compensation.

Arteriovenous Oxygen Difference

The arteriovenous oxygen difference is a measure of the amount of oxygen taken up from the blood by the tissues. Cardiac output and arteriovenous oxygen difference are the determinants of overall oxygen uptake. During exercise blood flow increases to the tissues; haemoglobin dissociates quicker and easier. This results in a greater arteriovenous oxygen difference during exercise. In trained athletes, the arteriovenous oxygen difference is greater as a result of the tissues becoming more efficient in oxygen uptake with aerobic training.

Thermoregulation During Exercise

The heat produced by the increase in metabolism during exercise must be dissipated in order to prevent a dangerous increase in core temperature. This is best accomplished by vasodilation of the blood vessels in the skin. This allows for the heated blood to pass close to the body surface and losing heat through radiation and conduction. The sweat glands is stimulated by the heated blood resulting in an increase in sweat production and thus losing more heat through evaporation. This evaporation of sweat leads to fluid and electrolyte loss, which can result in dehydration.

Dehydration may lead to impaired cognitive and exercise performance and heat stroke. Vasoconstriction happens at the viscera to maintain blood pressure in response to the fluid loss and redirection of blood to the skin.

Nervous System

Among the many functions of the nervous system is the control of movement by way of the skeletal muscles, which are under voluntary (and reflex) control. Most of the study of the neural control of movement is considered the domain of motor control and learning. However, certain areas of inquiry are also of interest to exercise physiologists. Two notable areas are neuromuscular fatigue and neurological adaptations to strength training. With respect to neuromuscular fatigue, research suggests that under certain conditions the Central Nervous System may play an important role in the development of fatigue. For example, changes in brain levels of serotonin and dopamine may influence fatigue. In addition, the firing rate of motor units can change during fatigue , which may be due to an elegant interplay between peripheral receptors and the CNS.

Similarly, strength training may influence the CNS control of muscle activation by changing the number of motor units that the CNS will activate during a contraction and the firing rate of the active muscle . Much of the data regarding neurological adaptations to strength training are contradictory, but this remains an important area of study. These areas of study are important to basic researchers in exercise physiology, and new information in these areas may also have implications in the rehabilitation of individuals with neuromuscular disorders.

The Autonomic Nervous System (ANS) is involved in the involuntary control of body functions. The ANS has two divisions. The Sympathetic Nervous System becomes active during situations of increased stress, such as during exercise. The Parasympathetic Nervous System is more active during resting conditions. Most notable in exercise physiology is the autonomic control of the cardiovascular system. For example, during exercise an increase in Sympathetic Activity and a decrease in Parasympathetic Activity result in an increase in activity of the heart and an increase in blood pressure. In addition, the ANS is involved in the redistribution of blood flow away from inactive tissues, such as the gastrointestinal tract, and toward the active tissues during exercise.

Endocrine System

The endocrine system is the system of hormones, which are chemicals released into the blood by certain types of glands called endocrine glands. Many hormones are important during exercise and may affect performance. For example, during exercise the hormone called growth hormone increases in concentration in the blood. This hormone is important in regulating blood glucose concentrations. Similarly, other hormones, such as cortisol, epinephrine, and testosterone, increase during exercise. Their effects may be short term in that they affect the body during the exercise bout. Other effects are prolonged and may be important in the long-term adaptation to regular exercise.

Adaptations to Exercise

Exercise training challenges many human physiological systems that need to adapt in order to maintain homeostasis, this is the inner balance of the body. While exercising, homeostasis is endangered by the increased amount of O_2 and nutrients demand, the need to get rid of $CO2$ and metabolic waste products, rising body temperature and acid imbalance and varying hormone levels.

Acute Adaptations to Exercise

Cardiovascular Responses

All the cardiovascular system components, heart, blood vessels and blood, are involved in the immediate response of the cardiovascular system to physical stress. During exercise, the cardiovascular response is largely directly proportional to the oxygen consumption of skeletal muscles.

Cardiac Output

Cardiac Output (Q) is defined as the amount of blood pumped by the left ventricle of the heart per minute. It is expressed as litres/minute. It is the product of heart rate (HR) X stroke volume (SV).

A person's maximum oxygen uptake ($VO_{2\,max}$) is the cardiac output (Q) X arteriovenous oxygen difference (A-VO_2).

The arteriovenous difference is a measure for the oxygen intake from the blood as it passes the body, e.g. activated muscle cells. The unit is millimetres oxygen per 100 mL of blood. At rest the value is on average about 4-5 mL/100mL of blood and can raise progressively during an exercise up to 16 mL/100mL of blood (4).

Cardiac output multiplied with A-VO_2 difference form the maximum oxygen uptake capacity (VO_{2max}) of an individual.

With a stepping working rate, the cardiac output increases in a nearly linear fashion in order to meet the increasing oxygen demand.

Cardiac Output is Measured by Echocardiography

With increasing physical stress, blood flow is directed away from the internal organs to the activated muscles; at maximal rates of work, 80 percent of the cardiac output goes to the activated muscles and the skin, whereas in rest this value is just twenty percent.

Blood Pressure

There is a linear increase in systolic blood pressure to peak values of 200 to 249 mmHg in normotensive individuals, and the diastolic pressure value remains near rest level.

Hypertensive individuals reach higher systolic blood pressures at a given rate of work, and they can also reach higher diastolic values. The peripheral resistance of blood flow is related to vessel diameter and length and blood viscosity in the peripheral vessels. Under physical demands the vessels dilate, increasing their diameters. Hypertension patients have increased peripheral resistance compared to normal, and this is a major cause of their higher average blood pressure. Two to three hours post exercise blood pressure drops below pre-exercising values, this is known as "post exercise hypotension".

Coronary Circulation

Coronary arteries supply the myocardium with blood and nutrients; on average one capillary supplies one myocardial fibre in the ventricular walls and papillary muscles.

Pulmonary System Adaptations

Pulmonary ventilation is initiated via the respiratory centre in the brainstem with parallel activation through the motor cortical drive that activates skeletal muscles and afferent Type III-IV muscle afferent fibres.

While maximum exercise training ventilation rates in normal-sized healthy people may increase by a factor of ten, compared to ventilation rates at rest.

Resistance Exercise

Dynamic training and resistance training differ primarily in the fact that resistance training produces a vigorous increase in the peripheral vascular resistance.

In the case of resistance training, high isolated forces are generated in the activated musculature. The strong isolated muscle contraction compresses the small arteries and thus increases the peripheral vessel resistance.

Skeletal Muscle Fibre Type

The type of physical exercise being undertaken determines the predominant muscle fibre type.

Regular, longer-lasting endurance training increases the number of mitochondria and the gas exchange capacity of the trained myofibrils. In marathon runners slow-twitch fibres dominate the trained leg muscles, while sprinters possess predominantly fast-twitch fibres. Endurance training has the potential to change metabolic properties of skeletal muscles in the direction of an oxidative profile. The question as to how far muscle fibre types can be reprogrammed remains open.

Hormonal Responses to Exercise

The stress hormones adrenaline and noradrenaline (the catecholamines) are responsible for many physiological adaptation procedures through training. Catecholamines are part of cardiovascular and respiratory training adaptations, and in fuel mobilisation and utilisation.

Immunological Adjustments

Moderate training enhances some components of the immune system and thereby reduces the susceptibility to infections. In contrast, a reduced functionality of immune cells occurs after over-straining.

Chronic Adaptations of Exercise

Skeletal Muscle Adaptations to Endurance Training

Slow-twitch fibres: The cross-sectional area of slow-twitch (AKA red) fibres increases slightly in response to aerobic work.

Fast-twitch fibres: These fibres develop a higher oxygen capacity.

Capillary bed density: Trained muscles possess a higher density of capillaries than untrained muscle, which permits a greater blood flow with increased delivery of nutrients.

Resistance Training Adaptations in Skeletal Muscle Cells

Resistance training causes increased muscle size (hypertrophy) through an increase of myofibril size and number of fast- and slow-twitch fibres. Moreover the recruitment pathway of muscle fibres become more effective. Resistance training thus leads to a greater force development of the trained muscles.

Ligament and Tendon Adaptations

There is an increase in cross-sectional area of ligaments and tendons in response to prolonged training, as the insertion sites between ligaments and bones and tendons and bones become stronger.

Metabolic Adaptations of Prolonged Exercise

Endurance training increases the size and number of mitochondria in the trained muscle; the myoglobin content may sometimes increase, thus the oxygen storage capacity increases sometimes. In trained muscles glycogen storage capacity increases, and the ability to use fat as an energy source.

Long Term Cardiac Adaptations

When healthy individuals participate in a long term aerobic exercise programme they undergo positive cardiac adaptions, both morphologically and physiological. They have increased early diastolic filling and increased contractile strength. Morphological changes appear in both the left and the right ventricle. The cardiac adaptations lead to increased cardiac output while exercising, and a higher VO_{2max} after exercise.

Post-training heart rate is decreased at rest and during sub-maximal exercise. Stroke volume increases through long term endurance training. Endurance training increases plasma volume, which elevates the blood volume that returns to firstly the right heart and after that to the left ventricle. The greater amount of blood in circulation causes an increase in the amount of blood in the left ventricle when the end-diastolic phase is reached. The end-diastolic phase is the phase in which the passive filling (diastole) of the heart finishes. The left ventricle is fully filled and its wall is stretched. The passive stored energy in the wall helps to a forceful contraction in the emptying phase (systole). As a result, the heart muscle is hypertrophied. Each heart muscle fibre increases in size. The hypertrophy refers to the ventricle and the posterior and septal walls.

High blood pressure = systolic blood pressure ≥140 and/or diastolic blood pressure ≥90 mm Hg blood pressure. The positive correlation of blood pressure and cardiovascular disease (CVD) risk starts from 115 mm Hg systolic and 75 mm Hg diastolic and doubles with every 20 mm Hg systolic and 10 mm Hg diastolic increase. According to the American College of Sports medicine, dynamic aerobic training reduces blood pressure (BP) in individuals with hypertension. Hypertension is a risk factor for cardiovascular events. Endurance exercises lower arterial blood pressure for some hours after a bout of exercise, this phenomenon is the post-exercise hypotension. Post-exercise hypotension seems to be greater in people with higher pre-exercise blood pressure values.

Blood pressure reductions occur after short bouts of exercises of 3 minutes duration and an intensity of 40% VO_{2max}.

Morphological cardiac adaptations is less in people with cardio vascular disease than when compared to younger, healthy people.

Long Term Respiratory Adaptations

The blood flow in the upper regions of the lungs increases after prolonged endurance training and the respiration rate increases.

Absolute Contraindications to Exercise

- Unstable Cardiovascular Disease (peripheral and central): acute myocardial infarction or unstable angina until stable for at least 5 days, dyspnoea at rest, pericarditis, myocarditis, endocarditis, symptomatic aortic stenosis, cardiomyopathy, unstable or acute heart failure, uncontrolled tachycardia.

- Fever: should be settled to avoid a risk of developing myocarditis.

- Acute pulmonary embolism or pulmonary infarction. Excessive or unexplained breathlessness on exertion.

- Any acute severe illness.

- Serious musculoskeletal injury/problem.

- Severely impaired cognitive functioning .

Precautions with Exercise

- Uncontrolled or poorly controlled asthma.

- COPD: Patients are required to be stable before training and oxygen saturation levels should be above 88-90%.

- Cancer or blood disorders: when treatment or disease cause leukocytes below 0.5 x109/L, haemoglobin below 60g/L or platelets below 20 x 109/L. If a patient has a platelet count of <20 000 then only AROM and ADLs are adviced due to the increased risk of bleeding, 20 000-30 000: light exercise only.

- Diabetes: If blood glucose is >13 mmol or <5.5 mmol/l then it should be corrected first.8 Patients with severe diabetic peripheral or autonomic neuropathy or foot ulcers should be assessed before undertaking exercise. Cease exercise with diabetes with acute illness or infection.

- Hypertension: resting blood pressures of a systolic >180 or diastolic >100 or higher should receive medication before regular physical activity with particular restrictions on heavy weights strength conditioning, which can create particularly high pressures.

- Osteoporosis: avoid activities with a high risk of falling.

- Unexplained dizzy spells.

Adverse Effects

Musculoskeletal Adverse Effects

Sudden force development, or repetitive movements can lead to musculoskeletal strain, tear or fracture.

Cardiovascular Events

In an epidemiological study, Prevalence of Sudden Cardiac Arrest (SCA) was studied between 2002-2013 and was compared with medical data in the USA. Of 1,247 cases of SCA, 63 were occurred during sport activities. The affected persons were 51.1 ±8.8 years old. The incidence is 21.7 (95% -CI 8.1-35.4) per million per year and varies based on sex for sports SCA. Men possess a Risk Ratio of 2.58 (95%-CI 2.12-3.13).

Another study investigated the Sudden Death in Athletes. They found a total of 2406 deaths between years 1980-2011. The young athletes were 19 ±6 years old and were engaged in 29 diverse sports. Young men were affected 6.5 times more frequently than women. The most common reason was hypertrophic cardiomyopathy.

Sports Physiology

Sports physiology is the study of the long-and short-term effects of training and conditions on athletes. This specialized field of study goes hand in hand with human anatomy. Anatomy is about structure, where physiology is about function.

Sports Training Principles are heavily rooted in this field. Effects of body composition, flexibility training, hydration, environmental conditions, and carbohydrate loading on athletic performance are only a few of the topics explored in this field.

Exercise physiologists, physicians, and athletic trainers can apply research findings from studies to advise athletes on topics concerning nutrition, sport-related injuries, and other issues related to sports medicine.

Understanding the internal effects of exercise on athletes sets the stage for designing fitness training programs that prepare them for the physical demands of specific sports. Don't forget, though, that internal changes in athletes' bodies are one piece of the training puzzle.

It is important to know that in order to understand the effects of training, scientists must "zoom in" under lab conditions. Athletes and coaches must consider how well artificial conditions apply to training athletes in the real world. Be careful not to take theories (possible explanations) as the "gospel" when training athletes--always "zoom out" into the real world of competition.

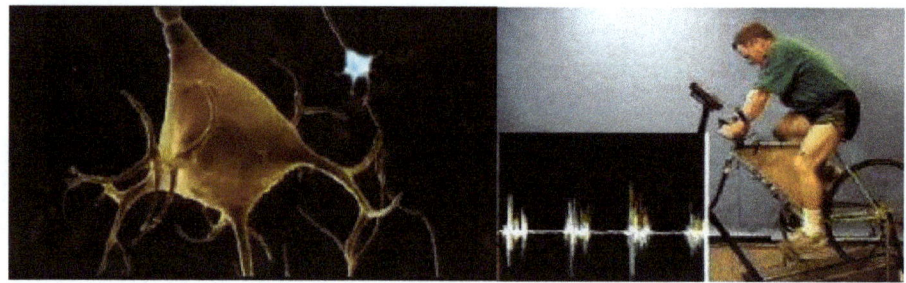

The best coaches read a variety of professional and scholarly resources in the field from publications such as the American Journal of Sports Medicine, the Journal of Strength and Conditioning Research, and the Journal of Sport Sciences. After reading the research, practitioners then consider how applications from each study fit with those from other sport sciences, and temper research findings with personal experience and good judgment.

References

- Exercise-physical-fitness: britannica.com, Retrieved 31 March, 2019

- Best-agility-drills-for-athletes: verywellfit.com, Retrieved 14 July, 2019

- Physiology-in-sport: physio-pedia.com, Retrieved 19 April, 2019

- Exercise-physiology: physio-pedia.com, Retrieved 17 May, 2019

- Sportsphysiology: sports-training-adviser.com, Retrieved 5 February, 2019

2
Optimal Nutrition for Exercise

Optimal nutrition is necessary to supply the nutrient for tissue maintenance, repair and growth. Energy and nutrients mainly come from three macronutrients, namely, carbohydrates, proteins and fats. This chapter closely examines these macronutrients to provide an extensive understanding of the subject.

Protein

Protein is also important for health and physical activity. The main role of protein in the body is for growth, repair and maintenance of body cells and tissues, such as muscle.

Different foods contain different amounts and different combinations of amino acids (the building blocks of proteins). Essential amino acids are those that the body cannot make itself and so are needed from the diet. The full range of essential amino acids needed by the body (high protein quality) is found in:

- Animal sources – meat, fish, eggs, milk, cheese and yogurt.

- Plant sources – soy, tofu, quinoa and mycoprotein e.g. Quorn.

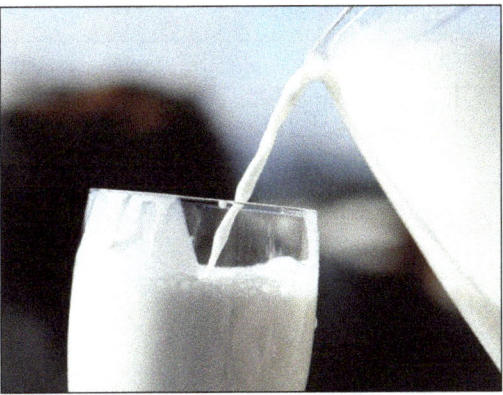

As some high protein foods can also be high in saturated fat, it is important to choose lower fat options, such as lean meats or lower fat versions of dairy foods.

Most vegans get enough protein from their diets, but it is important to consume a variety of plant proteins to ensure enough essential amino acids are included.

The protein requirements of a normal adult are 0.75g per kilogram of body weight per day. For strength and endurance athletes, protein requirements are increased to around 1.2-1.7g of protein per kilogram of bodyweight per day. If you are participating in regular sport and exercise like swimming/running or go to the gym on a regular basis, then your protein requirements may be slightly higher than the general sedentary population, in order to promote muscle tissue growth and repair. However, most people in the UK consume more than the recommended amount of protein, so increasing your protein intake is generally unnecessary.

Consuming a healthy, varied diet containing nutrient dense foods will ensure you get enough protein without the use of protein supplements or special high-protein eating strategies, even if your needs are a little higher! But try and spread your protein intake throughout the day.

It is a common myth that consuming lots of extra protein gives people bigger muscles. Quite often, people taking part in exercise focus on eating lots of protein, and consequently may not get enough carbohydrate, which is the most important source of energy for exercise. A modest 20g of high quality protein, equivalent to approximately half of a medium sized grilled chicken breast or a small can of tuna, has been shown to be enough for optimum muscle protein synthesis following any exercise or training session. Any more protein than this will not be used for muscle building and just used as energy.

As well as including protein as part of a healthy, balanced diet, the incorporation of some protein after exercise is important for building new muscle tissues and repairing the damaged ones.

The table below shows the protein content of some common foods:

Food source	Serving size	Protein content (g) per serving size
Chicken breast grilled	Medium (130g)	42
Salmon fillet grilled	Large (170g)	42
Rump steak grilled	115g (5oz)	36
Tuna canned in brine	Small can (100g)	25
Baked beans	1 can (415g)	22
Almonds	100g	21
Haddock grilled	Medium (85g)	20
Eggs	2 average size eggs (100g)	13
Lentil soup	1 can (400g)	12
Half fat cheddar cheese	4 tbsp grated (40g)	11
Low fat milk	300ml	10
Greek style plain yogurt	Small pot (120g)	7
Low fat fruit yogurt	Small pot (120g)	7

Carbohydrates

- Body carbohydrate stores provide an important fuel source for the brain and muscle during exercise, and can be manipulated by exercise and dietary intake.

- A key strategy in promoting optimal performance in competitive events or training is modifying the timing, amount and type of carbohydrate food and drinks according to the demands of the session and the individual needs of the athlete.

- Different dietary approaches for optimal sporting performance, for example a 'low carbohydrate high fat' diet and carbohydrate 'periodization', continue to be explored. However, there is a need for additional and improved evidence to support their widespread use.

Maintaining an optimal diet has many benefits to athletes, including improved and consistent performance, enhanced recovery, maintaining ideal body weight and composition, and a reduced risk of injury. Whether a weekend warrior or professional athlete, carbohydrate rightfully receives a great deal of attention in sports nutrition.

Importance of carbohydrates for exercise:

Key Energy Source

Carbohydrates provide the body with its first option for energy and are a key fuel for the brain and central nervous system. During any type of activity, muscles use glucose from carbohydrate for fuel.

Easily Digestible

Carbohydrate foods are an easy option prior to exercise. They are generally well tolerated and preferred by athletes, with the ability to be more easily digested compared to fat or protein foods.

Versatile

Carbohydrates can support exercise over a range of intensities due to its use by both anaerobic and oxidative pathways. For short and high intensity exercise, muscle and liver stores of glycogen provide the main source of energy, which need to be replaced post training sessions. For longer exercise, the extent of carbohydrate utilisation varies depending on intensity, type of training and overall diet.

Strong Evidence to Support Carbohydrate Availability Improves Performance

Performance of prolonged, sustained or intermittent high-intensity exercise is enhanced by strategies that maintain high carbohydrate availability (i.e., matching glycogen stores and blood glucose to the fuel demands of exercise). In contrast, depletion of these stores is associated with fatigue in the form of reduced work rates, impaired skill and concentration, and increased perception of effort.

Easily Manipulated

The body's carbohydrate stores are relatively limited and can be acutely manipulated on a daily basis by dietary intake or even a single session of exercise to match the requirements of exercise.

Due to the above factors, the low availability of carbohydrate stores can play a major limiting factor for exercise performance. A key strategy in promoting optimal performance in competitive events or training is matching an athlete's carbohydrate stores with the fuel demands of the session, with a focus on dietary carbohydrate pre, during and post exercise. The amount of carbohydrate needs to be sufficient to fuel athletes' training programmes and optimise the recovery of muscle glycogen stores between workouts.

Carbohydrate requirements for activity:

Intensity level	Activity Example	Carbohydrate requirements	Timings
Light	Low intensity or skills-based activities – technical	3-5g/kg of athlete's body weight/d	• Timing of intake of carbohydrate over the day may be manipulated to promote high carbohydrate availability for a specific session by consuming carbohydrate before or during a session, or during recovery of a previous session.
Moderate	Moderate exercise programme (eg: 1h/d)	5-7g/kg/d	
High	Endurance program (e.g. 1-3h/d moderate to high intensity exercise).	6-10g/kg/d	
Very High	Extreme commitment (e.g. > 4-5h/d moderate to high intensity exercise).	8-12g/kg/d	• As long as the total fuel needs are provided, the pattern of intake may simply be guided by convenience, individual choice and sport rules.

Pre-exercise – Fueling

A carbohydrate rich meal or snack 1-2 hours prior to exercise can provide a good fuel source to meet the demands of general exercise. However, more rigorous fueling strategies are necessary prior to a competition or training session for some exercise modes, in order to provide high carbohydrate availability to maximise the training session and ensure fatigue does not reduce/shorten the session. For prolonged exercise (greater than 60 minutes), there is evidence consuming 1 to 4 g/kg carbohydrate in the 1-4 hours before exercise can enhance endurance and performance. In some circumstances there may be additional benefit from higher glycogen stores, achieved by carbohydrate loading. This protocol creates super compensation of muscle glycogen stores by following a higher carbohydrate diet (10-12g/kg every 24 hours) for 2-3 days leading up to an endurance event.

In general, foods with a low-fat, low fibre and low-moderate protein content are preferred for a pre-event meal as these are less likely to cause gastrointestinal issues. In athletes who experience pre-event nerves or those with uncertain timetables, a quickly digestible option may be beneficial, such as liquid meal supplements.

During Exercise - Performance

During shorter periods of exercise (less than 45 minutes), carbohydrate intake during exercise is not considered to be necessary. However, for longer periods there can be a number of performance benefits including glycogen sparing, provision of an exogenous muscle substrate, prevention of hypoglycaemia, delay hunger and activation of reward centres in the central nervous system. In addition, there is new evidence to suggest that "mouth sensing" (or mouth rinsing), which is the practice of providing frequent contact of carbohydrate to the mouth and oral cavity, can stimulate parts of the brain and central nervous system to enhance work output and pacing. The amount, type, and timing of carbohydrate depend on a number of factors including type of event, exercise and the athlete's preparation. A range of everyday foods, fluids and formulated sports products that include sports beverages may be used. However, it is important to ensure foods and fluids have been well tested by the athlete during training to avoid adverse gastrointestinal discomfort issues. In addition, ease of eating may be important in some sporting competitions. Removing foods from hard to open packaging may be beneficial to save time and avoid distraction.

Post Exercise – Recovery

The primary goal of post exercise carbohydrate recovery is glycogen restoration. Replacing carbohydrate is important between frequent bouts of exercise. Time plays an important factor in recovery as the rate of glycogen resynthesis is only 5% per hour, therefore an athlete should consume carbohydrate as soon as practical after the first workout. Approximately 1 to 1.2 g carbohydrate/kg/h during the first 4 - 6 hours has been proven to be effective in maximising refuelling time between workouts.

Carbohydrate-rich foods with a moderate to high glycemic index is recommended for a post-exercise meal as this provides the most readily available source of carbohydrate for muscle glycogen synthesis. A Post exercise meal containing a range of nutrients may assist in other recovery processes and the addition of protein can be beneficial particularly when carbohydrate intake is suboptimal or when frequent snacking is not possible, by promoting additional glycogen recovery .

Is there any Difference between Sucrose and Glucose on Exercise Performance?

Research to date suggests sucrose appears to be as effective as other highly metabolisable carbohydrates (e.g., glucose, glucose polymers) in providing an exogenous fuel source during endurance exercise, stimulating the synthesis of liver and muscle glycogen during exercise recovery and improving endurance exercise performance. While gaps exist in the understanding of the metabolic and performance consequences of sucrose ingestion before, during and after exercise relative to other carbohydrate types or blends, sucrose should continue to be regarded as one of a variety of options available to help athletes achieve their specific carbohydrate intake goals.

Is there any Benefit of a Low Carbohydrate High Fat diet for Athletes?

Low Carbohydrate High Fat (LCHF) diets have received a great deal of attention globally in recent years. Most of the discussion in LCHF diets for sports performance is based on enthusiastic claims and testimonials rather than a strong evidence base. Although adaptation to a LCHF (whether ketogenic or not) increases the muscle's capacity to utilise fat as an exercise substrate, there is no long-term evidence this leads to a clear performance advantage. In fact, there is a risk of impairing the capacity for high intensity exercise.

How does "Periodization" of Carbohydrate Intake Effect Performance?

There has been increasing interest in a "periodized" approach to carbohydrate availability in the training program, where sessions undertaken to promote adaptation are integrated with others focused on high quality performance outcomes. One such sequence of this periodized approach is the "sleep-low" strategy which consists of three stages; 1. A late afternoon high intensity session with high glycogen stores, 2. Withholding carbohydrate to maintain glycogen depletion during overnight recovery; and 3. A low-moderate intensity steady-state exercise session the following morning. One week of exposure to this strategy has been shown to be successful in improving performance in trained endurance athletes and could be implemented during the weeks preceding a competition before the taper period. Current research on this strategy has inherent limitations and as such, further studies are required to contribute to the evidence base.

The ability of diet to improve performance is an area of great interest, with continual emerging research. There is a need for ongoing research and practice to identify a range of approaches to optimal training and competition diets according to the specific requirements of an event and the experience of the individual. The provision of sufficient carbohydrate intake pre-, during and post exercise plays a crucial role in performance (in both training and competition).

Fat

Fat is an important component of a diet designed to fuel exercise. One gram of dietary fat equals nine calories and one pound of stored fat provides approximately 3,600 calories of energy. This calorie density (the highest of all nutrients), along with our seemingly unlimited storage capacity for fat, makes it our largest reserve of energy. While these calories are less accessible to athletes performing quick, intense efforts like sprinting or weight lifting, fat is essential for longer, slower, lower intensity and endurance exercise, such as easy cycling and walking.

Everything we eat is made up of macro and micronutrients that are converted to energy inside the body, helping to fuel all of our bodily functions.

Dietary fat has been blamed for many health problems, but it is actually an essential nutrient for optimal health. Adipose tissue (stored fat) provides cushion and insulation to internal organs, covers the nerves, moves vitamins (A, D, E, and K) throughout the body, and is the largest reserve of stored energy available for activity.

Stored body fat is different from dietary fat. Body fat is only stored in the body when we consume more calories than we use, from any and all foods we eat, not just from dietary fats. There is an optimal level of body fat for health and for athletic activity.

How the Body uses it

Fat provides the main fuel source for long-duration, low- to moderate-intensity exercise (think endurance sports such as marathons). Even during high-intensity exercise, where carbohydrate is the main fuel source, fat is needed to help access the stored carbohydrate (glycogen).

Using fat to fuel exercise, however, is dependent upon these important factors:

- Fat is slow to digest and be converted into a usable form of energy. (It can take up to six hours for this to occur.)

- After the body breaks down fat, it needs time to transport it to the working muscles before it can be used as energy.

- Converting stored body fat into energy takes a great deal of oxygen, so exercise intensity must decrease for this process to occur.

For these reasons, athletes need to carefully time when and how much fat they eat. In general, it's not a great idea to eat foods high in fat immediately before or during intense exercise. Aside from the fact that the workout will be done before the fat is available as usable energy, doing so can cause some uncomfortable gastrointestinal symptoms, such as nausea, vomiting, and diarrhea.

Popular Diets that use Fat as the Main Fuel Source

Popular low-carbohydrate and high-fat diets, such as the Ketogenic diet and Paleo diet, all work on the premise that lower carbohydrate intake, coupled with high fat and moderate to high protein intake leads to burning body fat as the main fuel source while exercising.

There is, in fact, some scientific evidence that shows long-term low-carb/high-fat diets to be safe and possibly helpful in improving metabolic risk factors for chronic disease. In studies, these diets have shown to be beneficial for performance in ultra-endurance sports while at least several months of adaptation to a low-carb/high-fat diet are required for metabolic changes to occur.

3
Aerobic Exercise

Aerobic exercise is a form of physical exercise which depends on the aerobic energy generating process for a low to high intensity workout. Some of its types are water aerobics, endurance training, cross training, etc. This chapter has been carefully written to provide an easy understanding of these components of aerobic exercise.

- Aerobic literally means "with oxygen", and refers to the use of oxygen in muscles' energy-generating process.

- Aerobic exercise includes any type of exercise, typically those performed at moderate levels of intensity for extended periods of time, that maintains an increased heart rate.

- In such exercise, oxygen is used to "burn" fats and glucose in order to produce adenosine triphosphate, the basic energy carrier for all cells.

- Initially during aerobic exercise, glycogen is broken down to produce glucose, but in its absence, fat metabolism is initiated instead.

- The latter is a slow process, and is accompanied by a decline in performance level.

- The switch to fat as fuel is a major cause of what marathon runners call "hitting the wall." There are various types of aerobic exercise.

- In general, aerobic exercise is one performed at a moderately high level of intensity over a long period of time.

- For example, running a long distance at a moderate pace is an aerobic exercise, but sprinting is not.

- Playing singles tennis, with near-continuous motion, is generally considered aerobic activity, while golf or doubles tennis, with their more frequent breaks, may not be.

Aerobic Respiration

Aerobic respiration is the process by which oxygen-breathing creatures turn fuel, such as fats and sugars, into energy.

Respiration is a process used by all cells to turn fuel, which contains stored energy, into a usable form. The product of respiration is a molecule called ATP, which can easily use the energy stored in its phosphate bonds to power chemical reactions the cell needs to survive.

Aerobic respiration is respiration that uses oxygen as a reactant. Aerobic respiration is much more efficient, and produces ATP much more quickly, than anaerobic respiration (respiration without oxygen). This is because oxygen is an excellent electron acceptor for the chemical reaction.

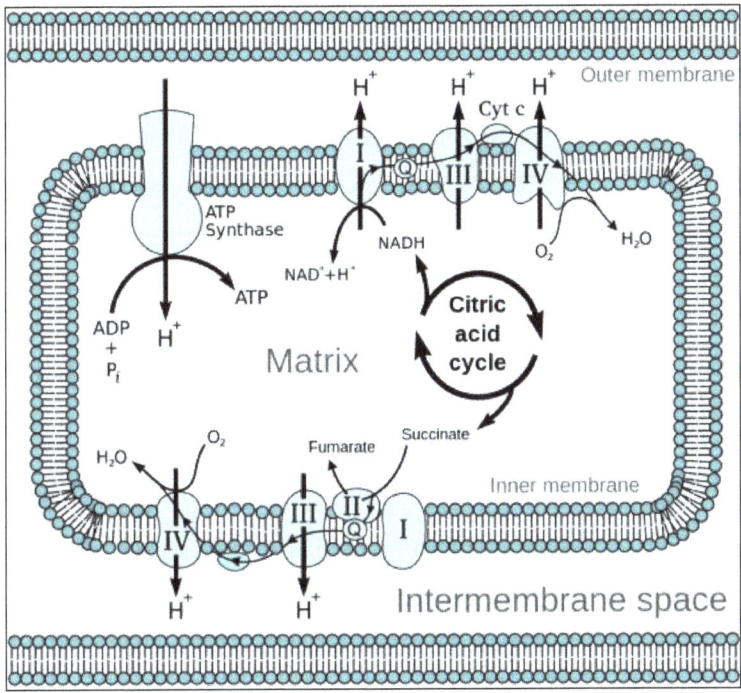

Common Steps Between Aerobic Respiration and Anaerobic Respiration

Both aerobic respiration and anaerobic respiration use an electron transport chain to move energy from its long-term storage in sugars to a more usable form.

In respiration, the energy from sugar is moved into ATP, which can be used to power many chemical reactions necessary to a cell's survival.

Both aerobic and anaerobic respiration start with the process of glycolysis. "Glycolysis," which literally means "sugar splitting," breaks a sugar molecule down into two smaller molecules.

In the process of glycolysis, two ATP molecules are consumed and four are produced. This results in a net gain of two ATP molecules produced for every sugar molecule broken down through glycolysis.

In cells that use oxygen, a sugar molecule is broken down into two molecules of pyruvate. In cells that do not have oxygen, the sugar molecule is broken down into other forms, such as lactate.

Although our cells normally use oxygen for respiration, which is much more efficient than anaerobic respiration, when we use ATP faster than we are getting oxygen molecules to our cells, our cells can perform anaerobic respiration to supply their needs for a few minutes.

After glycolysis, different respiration chemistries take a few different paths:

- Cells that are deprived of oxygen but are not made for anaerobic respiration, like our own muscle cells, may leave the end products of glycolysis sitting around, obtaining only two ATP per sugar molecule they split.

- Cells that are made for anaerobic respiration may continue the electron transfer chain to extract more energy from the end products of glycolysis.

- Cells using aerobic respiration continue their electron transfer chain in a highly efficient process that ends up yielding 38 molecules of ATP from every sugar molecule.

After glycolysis, cells that do not use oxygen may use a different electron acceptor, such as sulfate or nitrate, to drive their reaction forward.

These processes are called "fermentation." Some types of fermentation reactions actually have alcohol as their end product. So now you know where alcoholic drinks come from: the respiration processes of yeasts splitting sugars to produce energy.

Aerobic respiration, on the other hand, sends the pyruvate left over from glycolysis down a very different chemical path.

Aerobic Respiration and Weight Loss

Aerobic respiration is the process by which many cells, including our own, produce energy using food and oxygen. It also gives rise to carbon dioxide, which our bodies must then get rid of.

This equation explains why we need both food and oxygen, as both are reacted together to produce the ATP that allows our cells to function.

This equation also explains why we breathe out carbon dioxide – and how we lose weight.

This is also why you breathe harder and faster while performing calorie-burning activities: your body is using both oxygen and food at a faster-than-normal rate, and is producing more ATP to power your cells, along with more CO_2 waste product, as a result.

Unfortunately, simply breathing faster doesn't mean you'll unload more carbon: to lose carbon faster, your cells need to be consuming energy at a faster-than-normal rate. So get out those running shoes.

Aerobic Respiration Equation

The equation for aerobic respiration describes the reactants and products of all of its steps, including glycolysis. That equation is:

$$1 \text{ Glucose} + 6 O_2 \rightarrow 6 CO_2 + 6 H_2O + 38 \text{ ATP}$$

The reactions of aerobic respiration can be broken down into four stages, described below:

1. Glycolysis. In aerobic cells, the equation for glycolysis is:

$$\text{Glucose} + 2 HPO_4^{2-} + 2 ADP^{3-} + 2 NAD^+ \rightarrow 2 \text{ Pyruvate}^- + 2 ATP^{4-} + 2 NADH + 2 H^+ + 2 H_2O$$

Glycolysis in aerobic respiration refers to the splitting of a sugar molecule into two pyruvate molecules. This process creates two ATP molecules.

You will notice that this process also creates NADH from NAD^+. This is important because later in the process of cellular respiration, NADH will power the formation of much more ATP through the mitochondria's electron transport chain.

Pyruvate is then processed to turn it into fuel for the citric acid cycle, using the process of oxidative decarboxylation.

2. Oxidative decarboxylation of pyruvate

$$2\,(\text{Pyruvate}^- + \text{Conzyme A} + NAD^+ \rightarrow \text{Acetyl CoA} + CO_2 + \text{NADH})$$

In this process, pyruvate is combined with coenzyme A to produce acetyl-CoA.

You will note that more NADH is created in this step. This means more fuel to create more ATP later in the process of cellular respiration.

This is important because acetyl-CoA is an ideal fuel for the citric acid cycle, which can in turn power the process of oxidative phosphorylation *in the mitochondria, whic*h produces huge amounts of ATP.

3. Citric acid cycle

$$2\,(\text{Acetyl CoA} + 3\,NAD^+ + FAD + GDP^{3-} + HPO_4^{2-} + 2\,H_2O \rightarrow 2\,CO_2 + 3\,NADH + FADH_2$$
$$+ GTP^{4-} + 2\,H^+ + \text{Coenzyme A})$$

In the citric acid cycle, both NADH and $FADH_2$ – another carrier of electrons for the electron transport chain – are created. All the NADH and $FADH_2$ created in the preceding steps now come into play in the process of oxidative phosphorylation.

4. Oxidative phosphorylation

$$34\,(ADP^{3-} + HPO_4^{2-} + NADH + 1/2\,O_2 + 2\,H^+ \rightarrow ATP^{4-} + NAD^+ + 2\,H_2O)$$

Oxidative phosphorylation uses the folded membranes within the cell's mitochondria to produce huge amounts of ATP.

In this process, NADH and $FADH_2$ donate the electrons they obtained from glucose during the previous steps of cellular respiration to the electron transport chain in the mitochondria's membrane.

The electron transport chain consists of a number of complexes in the mitochondrial membrane, including complex I, Q, complex III, cytochrome C, and complex IV.

All of these ultimately serve to pass electrons from higher to lower energy levels, harvesting bits of their energy in the process. This energy is used to power proton pumps, which in turn power ATP formation.

Just like the sodium-potassium pump of the cell membrane, the proton pumps of the mitochondrial membrane are used to create a concentration gradient *which can be used to power other processes.*

In the case of the mitochondria's proton gradient, the protons that are transported across the membrane using the energy harvested from NADH and $FADH_2$ "want" to pass through channel proteins from their area of high concentration to their area of low concentration.

These channel proteins are actually ATP synthase – the enzyme that makes ATP. When protons pass through ATP synthase, they drive the formation of ATP.

This process is why mitochondria are referred to as "the powerhouses of the cell." The mitochondria's electron transport chain makes nearly 90% of all the ATP produced by the cell from breaking down food.

This is also the process that requires oxygen. Without oxygen molecules to accept the depleted electrons at the end of the electron transport chain, the electrons would back up and the process of ATP creation would not be able to continue.

Function of Aerobic Respiration

Aerobic respiration produces ATP, which is then used to power other life-sustaining functions, such as the action of the sodium-potassium pump, which allows us to move, think, and perceive the world around us; the actions of many enzymes; and the actions of countless other proteins that sustain life.

Complete Glucose Breakdown

The complete glucose breakdown is a series of chemical reactions representing transformation of glucose to adenosine triphosphate during the normal phases of aerobic cellular respiration. It is mostly done inside the mitochondria to release the maximum amount of energy.

Pyruvate is made from glucose during the glycolysis and transformed to an acetyl group during transition reaction. Glycolysis consists of ten enzymatic steps that occur in the cytoplasm of the cell. Glucose is converted to glucose-6-phosphate by hexokinase. This first step in the conversion of glucose to glucose-6-phosphate is a regulated step in glycolysis in which one ATP is used. From this phosphorylation, glucose in now trapped inside of the cell due to the negative charge from the phosphate group. Glucose-6-phosphate is converted to fructose-6-phosphate by phosphoglucoisomerase. Then, fructose-6-phosphate is converted to fructose-1,6-bisphosphate by phosphofructokinase. The use of the enzyme phosphofructokinase is the committed step which is under the greatest control for glycolysis. Fructose-1,6-bisphosphate is then converted to dihydroxyacetone phosphate (DHAP) and glycelaldehyde-3-phosphate (G3P) via aldolase. Next the DHAP is converted to G3P via triose phosphate isomerase. The two G3P now each are catalyzed by glyceraldehyde-3-phosphate dehydrogenase to produce two 1,3-bisphosphoglycerate. The two products then react with phosphoglycerate kinase to produce two 3-phosphoglycerate which then reacts with phosphoglycerate mutase to get two 2-phosphoglycerate. The two products then undergo an enolase reaction to get two phosphoenol pyruvate, which then reacts with pyruvate kinase to yield two pyruvate molecules. Pyruvate kinase is the last step of glycolysis and is irreversible. A phosphate group is transferred from phosphoenol pyruvate to ADP which produces a pyruvate and ATP. The pyruvates then undergo pyruvate oxidation to yield acetyl-CoA. The acetyl group is used in the Krebs cycle and the phase ends with the electron transport chain. During this stage, electrons are passed down the electron transport chain. Energy is released and captured for ATP production. The net result of this step is 34 ATP molecules

Benefits of Aerobic Exercise

The benefits of aerobic exercise can be broadly categorised as either 'fitness' (physical capacity) or 'health'. Fitness and health are linked, and most forms of aerobic exercise will help you achieve both.

Fitness — Including Increased Cardiorespiratory Fitness and Endurance (Stamina)

Regular aerobic exercise improves your cardiovascular fitness by increasing your capacity to use oxygen. It does this by increasing your heart's capacity to send blood (and hence oxygen) to the muscles. This is mainly achieved through an increase in the size of the heart's pumping chambers (ventricles), which means that your heart doesn't have to beat as fast to deliver the same amount of blood. This is evident in a slower resting heart rate, and a slower heart rate for the same exercise intensity.

As you get 'fitter', particular activities (such as walking or jogging at a specified speed) will become easier.

You'll also be able to undertake the activity for longer (known as endurance), and/or at a higher intensity (e.g. jogging at a faster speed). The same applies to activities such as cycling or swimming, but it should be noted that fitness tends to be specific. So jogging will provide only limited benefits to your swimming fitness and vice versa. However, a side-benefit you may notice is that you also have increased stamina for the everyday activities of life, not just for exercise.

Other fitness improvements occur in the exercising muscles, and are specific to those muscles being used in the mode of exercise (e.g. walking, running, cycling, or swimming). These include an increased capacity for the muscles to take up and use the additional oxygen being delivered by the heart.

Reduced Risk of Certain Health Problems

Regular aerobic exercise has been shown to reduce the risk of heart disease, high blood pressure, type 2 diabetes, colon cancer and breast cancer. It can lower blood pressure and improve your blood cholesterol by reducing the levels of LDL-cholesterol (so-called 'bad' cholesterol) and increasing the amount of HDL-cholesterol (so-called 'good' cholesterol). It can also reduce anxiety, stress and depression, as well as instilling a general sense of well-being. Regular aerobic exercise has even been shown to have the potential to increase your lifespan.

Low-impact aerobic exercise such as swimming is valuable for improving general health and fitness in people who have arthritis or other conditions that limit their ability to do weight-bearing exercise.

Importantly, whereas fitness tends to be quite specific, many health benefits can be gained from any form of aerobic exercise. Additionally, the health gains can be achieved from relatively moderate amounts of exercise — moving from a lifestyle involving no exercise to one that involves some exercise can lead to substantial improvements in health.

Weight Control

Aerobic exercise burns up energy (calories). Regular sessions of 30 to 60 minutes of low to moderate intensity aerobic exercise (at around 55 to 70 per cent of maximum heart rate) can be an important part of a weight loss or weight management programme that is also mindful of the energy (calories) consumed as food.

However, many of the health benefits associated with aerobic exercise occur independently of weight loss. Evidence from large studies has shown that active, overweight people do not have a greater risk of many diseases than inactive people who are not overweight. From a health perspective, it is of course best to be both active and a healthy weight, but if weight reduction is a problem, it doesn't mean that the exercise is having no benefit.

Improved Bone and Muscle Health

Your risk of osteoporosis (excessive bone thinning as you age) can be reduced by regular weight-bearing aerobic exercise such as brisk walking.

By stimulating the growth of tiny blood vessels in your muscle tissues, aerobic exercise has also been shown to lessen the pain experienced by people who have fibromyalgia or chronic low back pain, as the oxygen supply to the muscles is improved and waste products are removed more efficiently.

Social Benefits

Regular aerobic exercise can have social benefits too, whether you walk with a friend, play tennis with workmates, or form a social cycling team. Exercising with friends can also be the most effective way of ensuring that you do it regularly.

Aerobic Exercise Precautions

As with any form of exercise, be aware of over-exercising, either by doing aerobic exercise too hard, for too long or too often. This approach can lead to injury, and abandoning of your fitness programme. Remember to build up gradually from your current activity level, and not to progress too rapidly. If you are new to regular aerobic exercise, several weeks of low to moderate intensity aerobic exercise are usually advised before introducing more vigorous aerobic exercise sessions.

If you have existing health problems, are at high risk of cardiovascular disease, or have muscle, bone or joint injuries, check with your doctor before undertaking an aerobic exercise programme. Also, men aged over 40 years and women aged over 50 years who have not exercised regularly in the recent past should check with a doctor before undertaking a programme of vigorous physical activity.

Biologic Basis of Aerobic Exercise

Oxygen Delivery

Breathing increases during aerobic exercise to bring oxygen into your body. Once inside your body the oxygen is (1) processed by the lungs, (2) transferred to the bloodstream where it is carried by red blood cells to the heart, and then (3) pumped by the heart to the exercising muscles via the circulatory system, where it is used by the muscle to produce energy.

Oxygen Consumption

"Oxygen consumption" describes the process of muscles extracting, or consuming, oxygen from the blood. Conditioned individuals have higher levels of oxygen consumption than deconditioned individuals ("couch potatoes") due to biological changes in the muscles from chronic exercise training. For example, a deconditioned individual might have a maximal oxygen consumption of 35 milliliters (ml) of oxygen per kilogram of body weight per minute (ml/kg/min), whereas an elite athlete may have a maximal oxygen consumption up to 92 ml/kg/min. Values like this are expressed as VO_2 (volume of oxygen consumed) and can be measured with special equipment in a laboratory.

Burning Fat

A higher percentage of fat is burned during aerobic exercise than during anaerobic exercise. Fat is denser than carbohydrate (fat has nine calories per gram and carbohydrate has four), and so it takes more oxygen to burn it. During aerobic exercise, more oxygen is delivered to the muscles than during anaerobic exercise, and so it follows that a higher percentage of fat is burned during aerobic exercise when more oxygen is available. When less oxygen is present, like during anaerobic exercise, a higher percentage of carbohydrate is burned.

Keep in mind that both fuels are almost always burned simultaneously, except during the most intense, short-term bursts of energy, like sprinting and weightlifting. It's the percentage of fat and carbohydrate burned that changes during a workout depending on the intensity, but you almost never burn just one exclusively. You burn fat while you're at rest, and you burn it during virtually every moment of exercise. It's a myth to think that it takes 20-30 minutes of exercise before your muscles start burning fat.

Water Aerobics

Water aerobics (waterobics, aquatic fitness, aquafitness, aquafit) is the performance of aerobic exercise in fairly shallow water such as in a swimming pool. Done mostly vertically and without swimming typically in waist deep or deeper water, it is a type of resistance training. Water aerobics is a form of aerobic exercise that requires water-immersed participants. Most water aerobics is in a group fitness class setting with a trained professional teaching for about an hour. The classes focus on aerobic endurance, resistance training, and creating an enjoyable atmosphere with music. Different forms of water aerobics include: aqua Zumba, water yoga, aqua aerobics, and aqua jog.

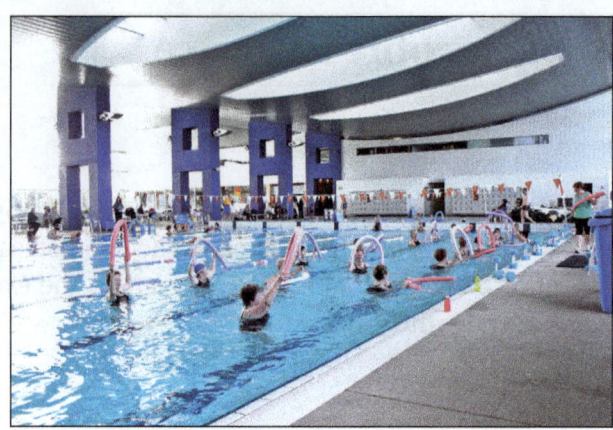
A water aerobics class at an Aquatic Centre.

Variation from Land-based Aerobics

While similar to land aerobics, in that it focuses on cardiac training, water aerobics differs in that it adds the component of water resistance and buoyancy. Although heart rate does not increase as much as in land-based aerobics, the heart is working just as hard and underwater exercise actually pumps more blood to the heart.

Exercising in the water is not only aerobic, but also strength-training oriented due to the water resistance. Moving your body through the water creates a resistance that will activate muscle groups. Hydro aerobics is a form of an aerobic exercise that requires water-immersed participants.

Variation of Format

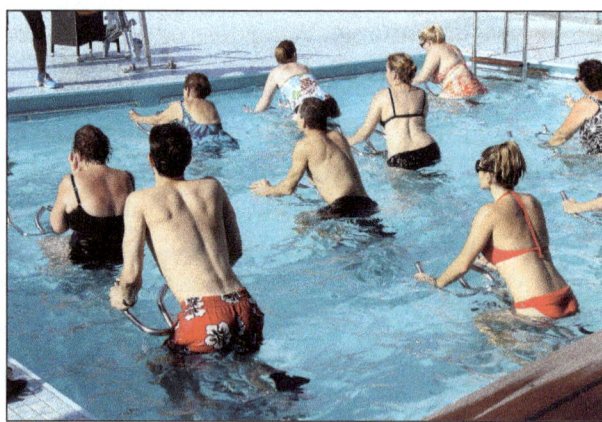
An Aqua cycling class.

New aquatic formats are arising into the exercise world with ideas such as: aqua cycling and water pole dancing. Water aerobics is beneficial to a multitude of participants because the density of the water allows easy mobility for those with arthritis, obesity, and other conditions. Further, it is an effective way for people of all ages to incorporate aerobics and muscle-strengthening into their weekly exercise schedule. Most classes last for 45–55 minutes. People do not even have to be strong swimmers to participate in water aerobics.

The performance of movement while suspended in water where the feet cannot touch the bottom surface, resulting in a non-impact, high-resistant, total body exercise workout, is known as deep water aerobics. Benefits of this method include less stress on the back, hips, knees and ankles.

Benefits

Most land-based aerobic exercisers do not incorporate strength training into their schedules and therefore adding aquatic exercise can greatly improve their health. As stated by the U.S. Department of Health and Human Services, "Adults should also [in addition to aerobic exercise] do muscle-strengthening activities that are moderate or high intensity and involve all major muscle groups on 2 or more days a week, as these activities provide additional health benefits." Over time water aerobics can lead to a reduction of blood pressure and resting heart rate, which will improve health overall.

According to Moreno and her quotes from Huey an Olympic athlete trainer, the benefits of water resistance training include the activation of opposing muscle groups for a balanced workout. The push and pull of the water allows both increased muscle training and a built-in safety barrier for joints. In fact, before water aerobics water, injury therapy used the benefits of water. The water also helps to reduce lactic acid buildup. Another obvious benefit to water exercise is the cooling effect of the water on the system. The average temperature around 78 degrees in a group fitness pool, this temperature will force the body to burn calories to stay at homeostasis while also maintaining a cool, comfortable atmosphere with less sweat noticeable to the participant.

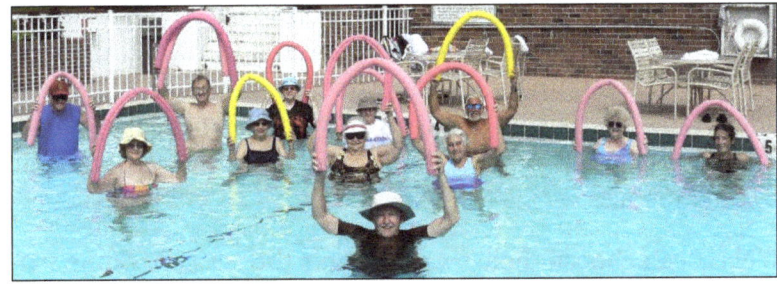
A water aerobics class incorporating flotation devices.

The mitigation of gravity makes water aerobics safe for individuals able to keep their heads out of water, including the elderly. Exercise in water can also prevent overheating through continuous cooling of the body. Older people are more prone to arthritis, osteoporosis, and weak joints therefore water aerobics is the safest form of exercise for these conditions. Research studies can teach us about the benefits the elderly can receive by participating in water aerobics. In a study done in Brazil, "Effects of water-based exercise in obese older women: Impact of short-term follow-up study on anthropometric, functional fitness and quality of life parameters" the effects of long-term water aerobics was tested. Although it did not conclude exactly as planned, their test subjects did experience improved aerobic capacity, muscle endurance, and better overall life quality. The water also provides a stable environment for elderly with less balance control and therefore prevents injury.

Disadvantages

Water aerobics has a few disadvantages from a practicality standpoint. Aqua aerobics requires access to a swimming pool via facilities, and in addition to any membership fees to access facilities, classes may cost extra. Although aquatic exercise greatly reduces the risk of injury, it is typically seen that not as many calories are burned as would be in some other activities. Though aquatic activities in general expend more energy than many land-based activities performed at the same pace due to the increased resistance of water, the speed with which movements can be performed is greatly reduced.

Indoor Cycling

Indoor cycling is a form of high-intensity exercise that involves using a stationary exercise bicycle in a classroom setting. The concept was created in the 1980s when Schwinn and ultra-endurance athlete Jonathan Goldberg ("Johnny G.") introduced the Spinning program. Participants set goals based on their heart rate, which can be measured by hand or using a heart rate monitor and rides simulate variations in terrain by altering resistance and cadence. If someone is new to indoor cycling and has not yet purchased a heart rate monitor then they can judge their level of exertion on an RPE (relative perceived exertion) scale. This scale has numbers which range from six (no exertion at all) to 20 (maximum exertion). Instructors will guide classes by mentioning what level of exertion a participant should be at.

A typical class involves a single instructor at the front of the class who leads the participants in a number of different types of cycling. The routines are designed to simulate terrain and situations encountered in actual bicycle rides, including hill climbs, sprints and interval training. Coasting downhill, obviously, is easiest to simulate. The instructor uses music and enthusiastic coaching to motivate the students to work harder. Most instructors will lead what is called an interval ride, this is where students will sprint, run, climb, and jump all in the same ride but there will not be definable pattern to the exercises.

Each person in the class can choose their own goals for the session. Some participants choose to maintain a moderate, aerobic intensity level, while others drive their heart rates higher in intervals of anaerobic activity. Besides being a great form of aerobic activity (burning between 400-600 calories in 40 minutes), spinning is also beneficial in strengthening the muscles of the lower body. It tones the quadriceps and hamstrings, along with working the back and hips. It can be difficult to stay at the moderate level in a class that is geared towards more intensity. If the exercise is not done correctly, injuries can occur; problems with the lower back and knees are most common. To avoid injury it is important to make sure the seat position is right for the participant's height. The seat should be set at a height such that the leg is fully extended with the foot resting on the pedal. Handlebar height can be adjusted for comfort; less experienced rider may want to set them higher to ease lower back discomfort.

Classes generally use specialized stationary bicycles. Features include a mechanical device to modify the difficulty of pedaling, specially-shaped handlebars, and multiple adjustment points to fit the bicycle to a range of riders. Many have a weighted flywheel which simulates the effects of inertia and momentum when riding a real bicycle. The pedals are equipped with toe clips as on sports bicycles to allow one foot to pull up when the other is pushing down. They may alternatively have clipless receptacles for use with cleated cycling shoes. Stationary cycles used in classroom settings often do not have the electronic features found on some models.

The difficulty of the workout is modulated in three ways:

- By varying the resistance on a flywheel attached to the pedals. The resistance is controlled by a knob, wheel or lever that the rider operates, causing the flywheel brake (a common bicycle brake, a friction wheel, a magnetic eddy-current brake, a viscoelastic fluid brake, or a strap running around the flywheel) to tighten. On most bikes the brake can be adjusted from completely loose, providing no resistance to pedaling beyond the inertia of the fly-wheel, to so tight that the rider can not move the pedals. Usually riders who can not pedal at the resistance called out by the instructor are encouraged to ride at a level at which they feel comfortable yet challenged.

- By changing the cadence (the speed at which the pedals turn). Pedaling slower against high resistance expends more energy than pedaling faster against low resistance.

- By sitting or standing in various positions:

  ◦ Forward, with hands at the front-most part of the handlebars where the handles are parallel to the sides of the rider's body, used only when out of the saddle.

  ◦ Middle, with hands on the 12-14" part of the handlebars that crosses the rider's body.

  ◦ Rear, with hands at the center part of the handlebars.

Each of these positions works the muscles in slightly different ways. Proper form for standing while pedaling requires the body to be more upright and the back of the legs touching or enveloping the point of the saddle, with the center of gravity directly over the crank. The center of gravity or pressure of body weight should never rest on the handlebars.

The three positions used in indoor cycling each work a different part of the body and it depends on the level of exertion whether or not someone changes position or the instructor can tell the class to change. Position one is when the rider in the saddle (seated) and the handles are resting on the center of the handle bars. Position two is when the rider stands up but can still feel the saddle between their legs and their hands are light on the handle bars because they are only there for balance. Position three is used for heavy climbing and the body is extended over the handles. It is important to remember to always be light on the handle bars because they are only there to help one balance and to adjust resistance accordingly when changing positions otherwise one's feet might stick in the pedals.

Most indoor cycling classes are coached with music. Riders may synchronize their pedaling to be in time with the rhythm of the music, thus providing an external stimulus to encourage a certain tempo. Often, the music chosen by the instructor is dance music or rock music set to a dance beat (i.e. 4/4 time), but not necessarily. This tends to help motivate participants to work harder than they might otherwise. The instructor also may choose specific song for sprints, climbs, and jumps. While the music provides a tempo cue, the cadence does not need to be a multiple of the beat in order for the rider to feel in rhythm; the music therefore helps a rider maintain any constant cadence, not just a cadence that matches the beat.

It is recommended when riding in a class to bring plenty of water. Indoor cycling is very energetic and causes a lot of sweating, and a person who is near dehydration can easily be dehydrated by the end of an hour of hard riding. One ounce (30 milliliters) of water consumed for each minute of work is the recommended and safest hydration ratio, but this could be varied depending on your weight.

The flywheel resistance control is also used to brake the flywheel. When changing from fast pedaling to slow, the flywheel brake may be used to slow the flywheel rather than allowing the force of the angular momentum to be applied to ones knees and legs.

Spinning as a Bicycling Technique

Spinning on a mobile bicycle refers to the technique of using a range of gears to maintain a constant rapid cadence of 60-110 rpm in controlled, even pedal strokes. This technique is recommended to improve bicycle control, aerobic fitness and endurance.

Aerobics

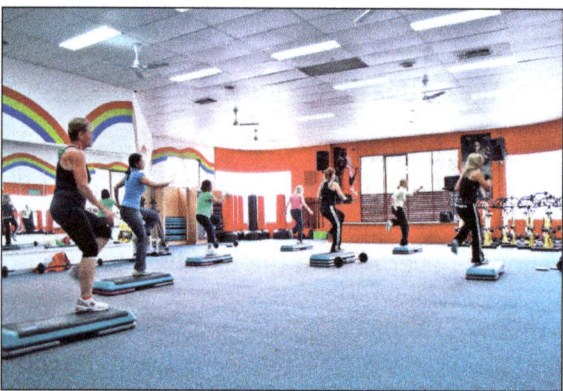
Step aerobics in a gym.

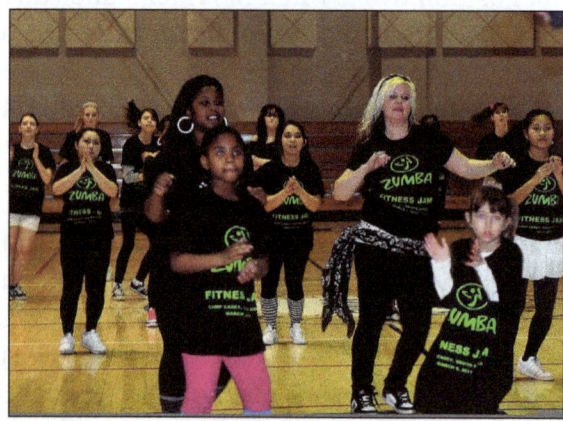
A dance aerobics class.

Aerobics is a form of physical exercise that combines rhythmic aerobic exercise with stretching and strength training routines with the goal of improving all elements of fitness (flexibility, muscular strength, and cardio-vascular fitness). It is usually performed to music and may be practiced in a group setting led by an instructor (fitness professional), although it can be done solo and without musical accompaniment. With the goal of preventing illness and promoting physical fitness, practitioners perform various routines comprising a number of different dance-like exercises. Formal aerobics classes are divided into different levels of intensity and complexity and will have five components: warm-up (5–10 minutes), cardiovascular conditioning (25–30 minutes), muscular strength and conditioning (10–15 minutes), cool-down (5–8 minutes) and stretching and flexibility (5–8 minutes). Aerobics classes may allow participants to select their level of participation according to their fitness level. Many gyms offer a variety of aerobic classes. Each class is designed for a certain level of experience and taught by a certified instructor with a specialty area related to their particular class.

Step Aerobics

Step aerobics is a form of aerobic exercise that uses a low elevated platform, the step, of height tailored to individual needs by inserting risers. Step aerobics classes are offered at many gyms.

Step aerobics was developed by Gin Miller around 1989. After a knee injury, Miller consulted with an orthopedic doctor, who recommended she strengthen the muscles supporting the knee by stepping up and down on a milk crate; from this she developed the step regimen.

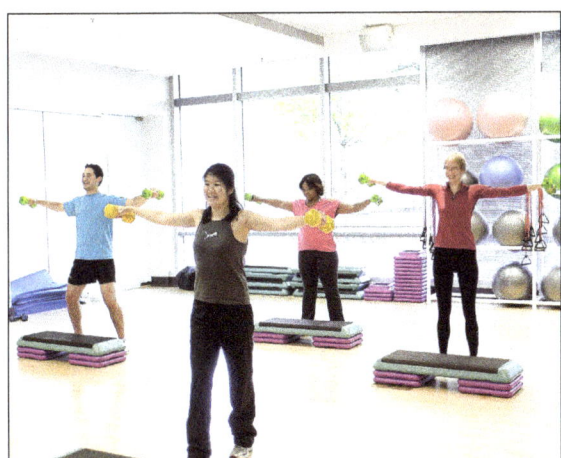
Aerobics using dumbells.

Step aerobics can also be involved in dancing games, such as Dance Dance Revolution or In the Groove.

Moves and Techniques

Often moves are referred to as Reebok step moves in reference to one of the first makers of the plastic step commonly used in gyms.

The "basic" step involves raising one foot onto the step, then the other so that they are both on the step, then stepping the first foot back, followed by the second. A "right basic" would involve stepping right foot up, then the left, then returning to the floor alternating right then left.

Some instructors switch immediately between different moves, for example between a right basic and a left basic without any intervening moves, effectively "tapping" the foot without shifting weight; tap-free or smooth stepping alternates the feet without "taps".

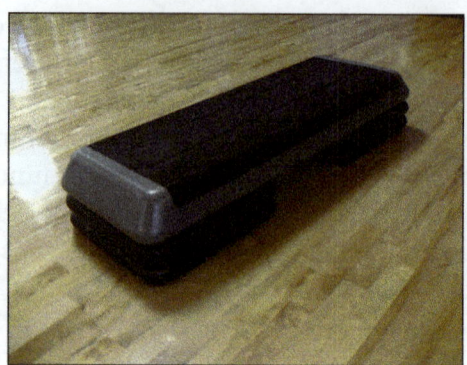

A step with 2 risers.

Common moves include:

- Basic Step

- Corner knee (or corner kick)

- Repeater knee (aka Triple knee)

- T-Step

- Over-the-Top

- Lunges

- V-Step

- Straddle Down

- L-Step

- Split Step

- I-Step

Choreography

Many instructors will prepare a set of moves that will be executed together to form the choreography of the class. Usually, the choreography will be timed to 32 beats in a set, ideally switching legs so that the set can be repeated in a mirrored fashion. A set may consist of many different moves and the different moves may have different durations. For example, a basic step as described above takes 4 beats (for the 4 steps the person takes). Similarly, the "knee up" move also takes 4 beats. Another common move, the repeater knee, is an 8-beat move.

Classes vary in the level of choreography. Basic level classes will tend to have a series of relatively basic moves strung together into a sequence. More advanced classes incorporate dance elements such as turns, mambos, and stomps. These elements are put together into 2–3 routines in each class. One learns the routines during the class and then all are performed at the end of the class. Regardless of the complexity of the choreography, most instructors offer various options for different levels of intensity/dance ability while teaching the routines.

Freestyle Aerobics

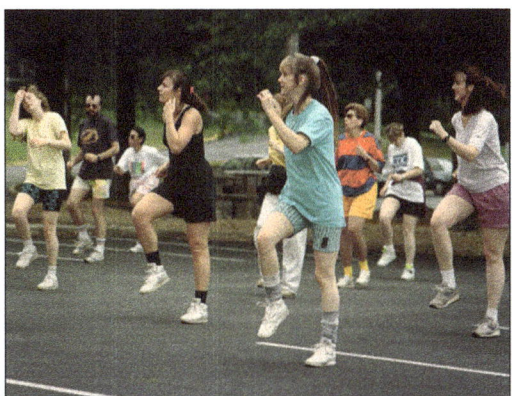
An aerobics class.

Freestyle aerobics is an aerobics style in which a group instructor choreographs several short dance combinations and teaches them to the class. This is usually achieved by teaching the class 1-2 movements at a time and repeating the movements until the class is able to join the whole choreography together. Aerobic music is used throughout the class. This is sometimes followed by a strength section which uses body weight exercises to strengthen muscles and a stretch routine to cool down and improve flexibility. Classes are usually 30–60 minutes in length and may include the use of equipment such as a barbell, aerobic step, or small weights.

In freestyle aerobics, the instructor choreographs the routine and adjusts it to the needs and wants of her/his class. There is often no difference between base movements in freestyle and pre-choreo-graphed programs.

It is practiced to improve aerobic fitness, flexibility and strength.

Aerobic Gymnastics

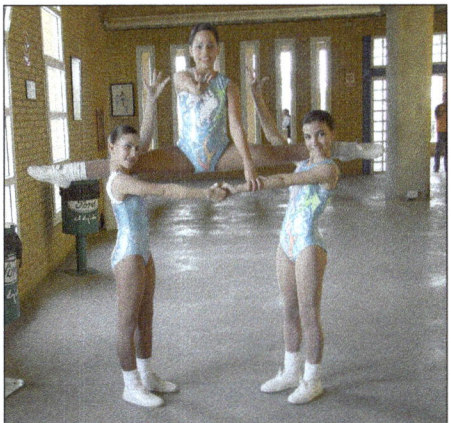
A sport aerobics team.

Aerobic gymnastics, also known as sport aerobics and competitive aerobics, may combine compli-cated choreography, rhythmic and acrobatic gymnastics with elements of aerobics. Performance is divided into categories by age, sex and groups (individual, mixed pairs and trios) and are judged on the following elements: dynamic and static strength, jumps and leaps, kicks, balance and flexibility.

Ten exercises are mandatory: four consecutive high leg kicks, patterns. A maximum of ten elements from following families are allowed: push-ups, supports and balances, kicks and splits, jumps and leaps. Elements of tumbling such as handsprings, handstands, back flips, and aerial somersaults are prohibited. Scoring is by judging of artistic quality, creativity, execution, and difficulty of routines. Sport aerobics has state, national, and international competitions, but is not an olympic sport.

Benefits

Like other forms of exercise, step aerobics helps burn calories and fat. The number of calories burned depends on the speed of movements, step height, length of exercise, and the persons height and weight.

Distance Running

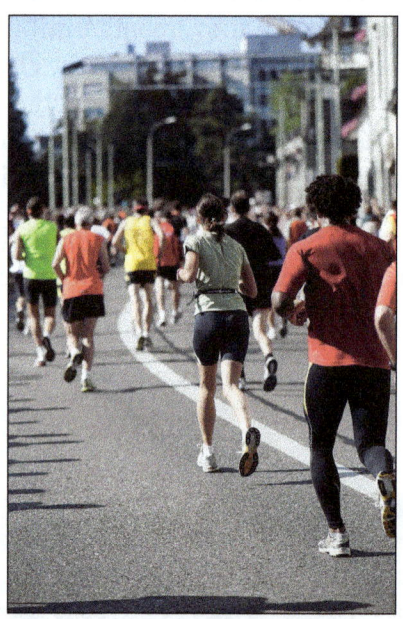

A group of amateur runners in a long-distance race in Switzerland.

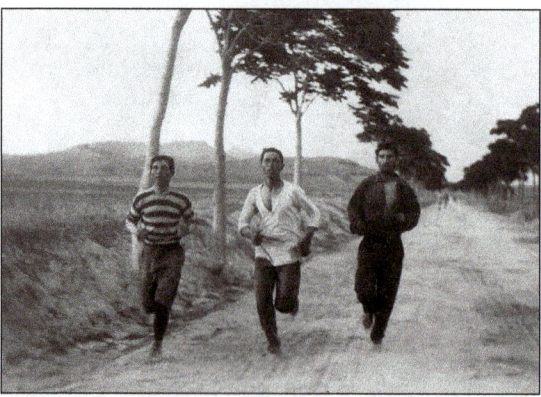

Burton Holmes' photograph entitled "1896: Three athletes in training for the marathon at the Olympic Games in Athens".

Long-distance running, or endurance running, is a form of continuous running over distances of at least 3 kilometres (1.8 miles). Physiologically, it is largely aerobic in nature and requires stamina as well as mental strength.

Among mammals, humans are well adapted for running significant distances, and particularly so among primates. The endurance running hypothesis suggests that running endurance in the genus *Homo* arose because travelling over large areas improved scavenging opportunities and allowed persistence hunting. The capacity for endurance running is also found in migratory ungulates and a limited number of terrestrial carnivores, such as bears, dogs, wolves and hyenas.

In modern human society, long-distance running has multiple purposes: people may engage in it for physical exercise, for recreation, as a means of travel, for economic reasons, or for cultural reasons. Long distance running can also be used as a means to improve cardiovascular health. Running improves aerobic fitness by increasing the activity of enzymes and hormones that stimulate the muscles and the heart to work more efficiently. Endurance running is often a component of physical military training and has been so historically. Professional running is most commonly found in the field of sports, although in pre-industrial times foot messengers would run to deliver information to distant locations. Long-distance running as a form of tradition or ceremony is known among the Hopi and Tarahumara people, among others. Distance running can also serve as a bonding exercise for family, friends, colleagues, and has even been associated with nation-building. The social element of distance running has been linked with improved performance.

In the sport of athletics, long-distance events are defined as races covering three kilometres (1.86 miles) and above. The three most common types are track running, road running and cross country running, all of which are defined by their terrain – all-weather tracks, roads and natural terrain, respectively. Typical long-distance track races range from 3000 metres to 10,000 metres (6.2 miles), cross country races usually cover 5 to 12 km (3 to 7½ miles), while road races can be significantly longer, reaching 100 kilometres (60 miles) and beyond. In collegiate cross country races in the United States, men race 8000 or 10000 meters, depending on their division, whereas women race 6000 meters . The Summer Olympics features three long-distance running events: the 5000 metres, 10,000 metres and marathon (42.195 kilometres, or 26 miles and 385 yards). Since the late 1980s, Kenyans, Moroccans and Ethiopians have dominated in major international long-distance competitions. The high altitude of these countries has been proven to help these runners achieve more success. Mountain air, combined with endurance training, can lead to an increase in red blood cells, allowing more oxygen to be passed through the veins. The majority of these East African successful runners come from three mountain districts that run along the Great Rift Valley.

Physiology of Long-distance Running

Humans are considered among the best distance runners among all running animals: game animals are faster over short distances, but they have less endurance than humans. Unlike other primates whose bodies are suited to walk on four legs or climb trees, the human body has evolved into upright walking and running around 2-3 million years ago. The human body can endure long distance running through the following attributes:

- Bone and muscle structure: unlike quadruped mammals, which have their center of mass in front of the hind legs or limbs, in biped mammals including humans the center of mass lies right above the legs. This leads to different bone and muscular demands especially in the legs and pelvis.

- Dissipation of metabolic heat: humans' ability to cool the body by sweating through the body surface provides many advantages over panting through the mouth or nose. These include a larger surface of evaporation and independence of the respiratory cycle.

One distinction between upright walking and running is energy consumption during locomotion. While walking, humans use about half the energy needed to run. Evolutionary biologists believe that the human ability to run over long distances has helped meat-eating humans to compete with other carnivores. Persistence hunting is a method in which hunters use a combination of running, walking, and tracking to pursue prey to the point of exhaustion. While humans can sweat to reduce body heat, their quadrupedal prey would need to slow from a gallop in order to pant.

Factors

Aerobic Capacity

One's aerobic capacity or VO_2Max is the ability to maximally take up and consume oxygen during exhaustive exercise. Long distance runners typically perform at around 75–85 % of peak aerobic capacity, while short distance runners perform at closer to 100% of peak.

Aerobic capacity depends on the transportation of large amounts of blood to and from the lungs to reach all tissues. This in turn is dependent on having a high cardiac output, sufficient levels of hemoglobin in blood, and an optimal vascular system to distribute of blood. A 20 fold increase of local blood flow within skeletal muscle is necessary for endurance athletes, like marathon runners, to meet their muscles' oxygen demands at maximal exercise that are up to 50 times greater than at rest.

Elite long distance runners often have larger hearts and decreased resting heart rates that enable them to achieve greater aerobic capacities. Increased dimensions of the heart enable an individual to achieve a greater stroke volume. A concomitant decrease in stroke volume occurs with the initial increase in heart rate at the onset of exercise. Despite an increase in cardiac dimensions, a marathoner's aerobic capacity is confined to this capped and ever decreasing heart rate.

The amount of oxygen that blood can carry depends on blood volume, which increases during a race, and the amount of hemoglobin in blood.

Other physiological factors affecting a marathon runner's aerobic capacity include pulmonary diffusion, mitochondria enzyme activity, and capillary density.

A long-distance runner's running economy is their steady state requirement for oxygen at specific speeds and helps explain differences in performance for runners with very similar aerobic capacities. This is often measured by the volume of oxygen consumed, either in liters or milliliters, per kilogram of body weight per minute (L/kg/min or mL/kg/min). As of 2016, the physiological basis for this was uncertain, but it seemed to depend on the cumulative years of running, and reaches a cap that longer individual training sessions cannot overcome.

Lactate Threshold

A long-distance runner's velocity at the lactate threshold is strongly correlated to their performance. Lactate threshold is the cross over point between predominantly aerobic energy usage and anaerobic energy usage and is considered a good indicator of the body's ability to efficiently process and transfer chemical energy into mechanical energy. For most runners, the aerobic zone doesn't begin until around 120 heart beats per minute. Lactate threshold training involves tempo workouts that are meant to build strength and speed, rather than improve the cardiovascular system's efficiency in absorbing and transporting oxygen. By running at your lactate threshold, your body will become more efficient at clearing lactic acid and reusing it to fuel your muscles. Uncertainty exists in regards to how lactate threshold affects endurance performance.

Fuel

In order to sustain high intensity running, a marathon runner must obtain sufficient glycogen stores. Glycogen can be found in the skeletal muscles or liver. With low levels of glycogen stores at the onset of the marathon, premature depletion of these stores can reduce performance or even prevent completion of the race. ATP production via aerobic pathways can further be limited by glycogen depletion. Free Fatty Acids serve as a sparing mechanism for glycogen stores. The artificial elevation of these fatty acids along with endurance training demonstrate a marathon runner's ability to sustain higher intensities for longer periods of time. The prolonged sustenance of running intensity is attributed to a high turnover rate of fatty acids that allows the runner to preserve glycogen stores later into the race.

Long distance runners generally practice carbohydrate loading in their training and race preparation.

Thermoregulation and Body Fluid Loss

The maintenance of core body temperature is crucial to a marathon runner's performance and health. An inability to reduce rising core body temperature can lead to hyperthermia. In order to reduce bodily heat, the metabolically produced heat needs to be removed from the body via sweating, which in turn requires re-hydration to compensate for. Replacement of fluid is limited but can help keep the body's internal temperatures cooler. Fluid replacement is physiologically challenging during exercise of this intensity due to the inefficient emptying of the stomach. Partial fluid replacement can serve to avoid a marathon runner's body over heating but not enough to keep pace with the loss of fluid via sweat evaporation. Environmental factors can especially complicate heat regulation.

Impact on Health

The impact of long-distance running on human health is generally positive. Various organs and systems in the human body are improved: bone mineral density is increased, cholesterol is lowered. However, beyond a certain point, negative consequences might occur. Male runners who run more than 40 miles (64 kilometers) per week face reduced testosterone levels, although they are still in the normal range. Running a marathon lowers testosterone levels by 50% in men, and more than doubles cortisol levels for 24 hours. Low testosterone is thought to be a physiological adaptation to the sport, as excess muscle caused may be shed through lower testosterone, yielding a more efficient runner. Veteran, lifelong endurance athletes have been found to have more heart scarring than controls groups, but replication studies and larger studies should be done to firmly establish the link, which may or may not be causal. Some studies find that running more than 20 miles (32 kilometers) per week yields no lower risk for all-cause mortality than non-runners, however these studies are in conflict with large studies that show longer lifespans for any increase in exercise volume.

The effectiveness of shoe inserts has been contested. Memory foam and similar shoe inserts may be comfortable, but they can make foot muscles weaker in the long term. Running shoes with special features, or lack thereof in the case of minimalist designs, do not prevent injury. Rather, comfortable shoes and standard running styles are safer.

In Sport

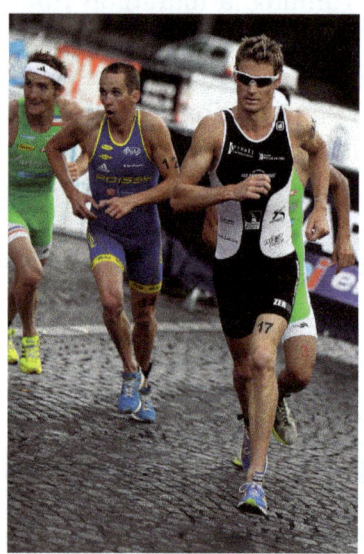

Men in the 10 km run section of the 2011 Grand Prix de Triathlon in Paris.

Many sporting activities feature significant levels of running under prolonged periods of play, especially during ball sports like association football and rugby league. However, continuous endurance running is exclusively found in racing sports. Most of these are individual sports, although team and relay forms also exist.

The most prominent long-distance running sports are grouped within the sport of athletics, where running competitions are held on strictly defined courses and the fastest runner to complete the distance wins. The foremost types are long-distance track running, road running and cross-country running. Both track and road races are usually timed, while cross country races are not always timed and typically only the placing is of importance. Other less popular variants such as fell running, trail running, mountain running and tower running combine the challenge of distance with a significant incline or change of elevation as part of the course.

Multisport races frequently include endurance running. Triathlon, as defined by the International Triathlon Union, may feature running sections ranging from five kilometres (3.1 mi) to the marathon distance (42.195 kilometres, or 26 miles and 385 yards), depending on the race type. The related sport of duathlon is a combination of cycling and distance running. Previous versions of the modern pentathlon incorporated a three or four kilometre (1.9–2.5 mi) run, but changes to the official rules in 2008 meant the running sections are now divided into three separate legs of one kilometre each (0.6 mi).

Depending on the rules and terrain, navigation sports such as foot orienteering and rogaining may contain periods of endurance running within the competition. Variants of adventure racing may also combine navigational skills and endurance running in this manner.

Track Running

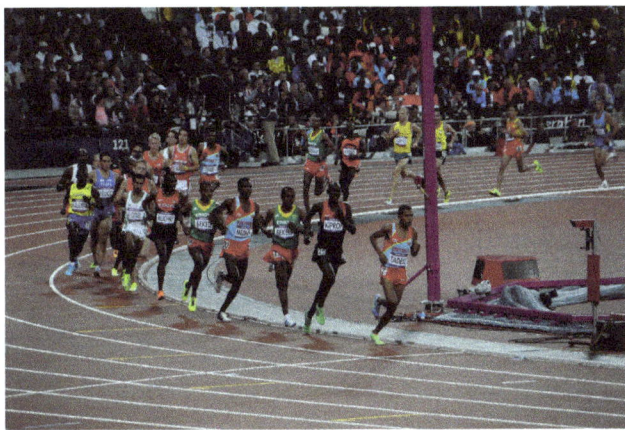

Runners turning the bend in the men's 10,000 metres final at the 2012 Summer Olympics.

The history of long-distance track running events is tied into the track and field stadia where they are held. Oval circuits allow athletes to cover long distances in a confined area. Early tracks were usually on flattened earth or were simply marked areas of grass. The style of running tracks became refined during the 20th century: the oval running tracks were standardised to 400 metres in distance and cinder tracks were replaced by synthetic all-weather running track of asphalt and rubber from the mid-1960s onwards. It was not until the 1912 Stockholm Olympics that the standard long-distance track events of 5000 metres and 10,000 metres were introduced.

- The 5000 metres is a premier event that requires tactics and superior aerobic conditioning. Training for such an event may consist of a total of 60–200 kilometers (40–120 miles) a week, although training regimens vary greatly. The 5000 is often a popular entry-level race for beginning runners:

  ○ The world record for men is 12:37.35 (an average of 23.76 km/h) by Kenenisa Bekele of Ethiopia in Hengelo, Netherlands on 31 May 2004.

  ○ The world record for women is 14:11.15 (an average of 21.14 km/h) by Tirunesh Dibaba of Ethiopia in Oslo, Norway on 6 June 2008.

- The 10,000 metres is the longest standard track event. Most of those running such races also compete in road races and cross country running events:

  ○ The world record for men is 26:17.53 (22.83 km/h) by Kenenisa Bekele of Ethiopia set in 2005.

- ◦ The world record for women is 29:17.45 (20.48 km/h) by Almaz Ayana of Ethiopia set on 12 August 2016.

- The one hour run is an endurance race that is rarely contested, except in pursuit of world records.

- The 20,000 metres is also rarely contested, most world records in the 20,000 metres have been set while in a one-hour run race.

Road Running

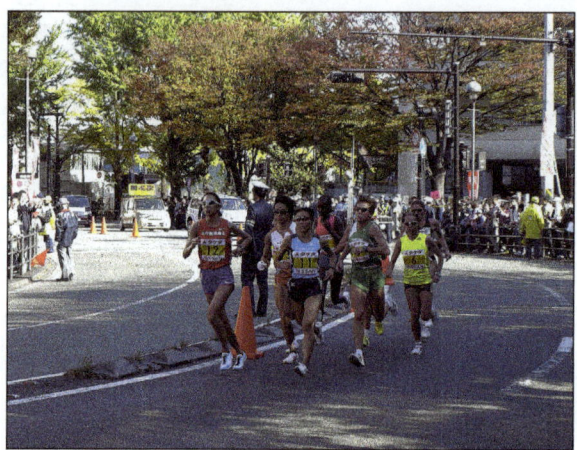

Women runners on a closed-off-road at the 2009 Yokohama Marathon.

Long-distance road running competitions are mainly conducted on courses of paved or tarmac roads, although major events often finish on the track of a main stadium. In addition to being a common recreational sport, the elite level of the sport – particularly marathon races – are one of the most popular aspects of athletics. Road racing events can be of virtually any distance, but the most common and well known are the marathon, half marathon and 10 km run.

The sport of road running finds its roots in the activities of footmen: male servants who ran alongside the carriages of aristocrats around the 18th century, and who also ran errands over distances for their masters. Foot racing competitions evolved from wagers between aristocrats, who pitted their footman against that of another aristocrat in order to determine a winner. The sport became professionalised as footmen were hired specifically on their athletic ability and began to devote their lives to training for the gambling events. The amateur sports movement in the late 19th century marginalised competitions based on the professional, gambling model. The 1896 Summer Olympics saw the birth of the modern marathon and the event led to the growth of road running competitions through annual public events such as the Boston Marathon (first held in 1897) and the Lake Biwa Marathon and Fukuoka Marathons, which were established in the 1940s. The 1970s running boom in the United States made road running a common pastime and also increased its popularity at the elite level.

The marathon is the only road running event featured at the IAAF World Championships in Athletics and the Summer Olympics, although there is also the IAAF World Half Marathon Championships held every two years. The marathon is also the only road running event featured at the IPC Athletics World Championships and the Summer Paralympics. The World Marathon Majors series includes the six most prestigious marathon competitions at the elite level – the Berlin, Boston, Chicago, London, Tokyo, and New York City marathons. The Tokyo Marathon was most recently added to the World Marathon Majors in 2012.

Ekiden contests – which originated in Japan and remain very popular there – are a relay race variation on the marathon, being in contrast to the typically individual sport of road running.

Cross Country Running

Cross country running is the most naturalistic form of long-distance running in athletics as competitions take place on open-air courses over surfaces such as grass, woodland trails, earth or mountains. In contrast to the relatively flat courses in track and road races, cross country usually incorporates obstacles such as muddy sections, logs and mounds of earth. As a result of these factors, weather can play an integral role in the racing conditions. Cross country is both an individual and team sport, as runners are judged on an individual basis and a points scoring method is used for teams. Competitions are typically races of 4 km (2.5 mi) or more which are usually held in autumn and winter. Cross country's most successful athletes often compete in long-distance track and road events as well.

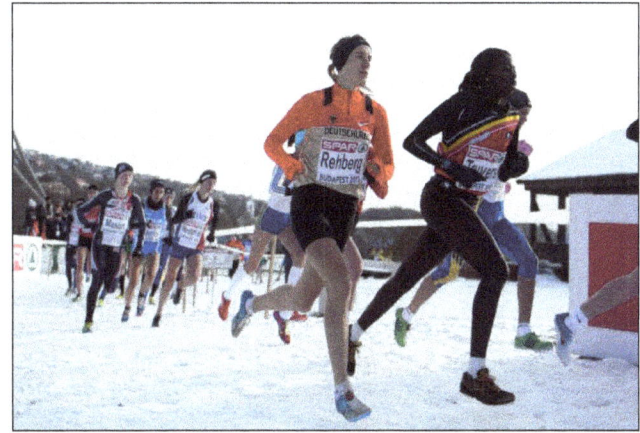

Women racing on snow in the 2012 European Cross Country Championships.

The history of the sport is linked with the game of paper chase, or hare and hounds, where a group of runners would cover long distances to chase a leading runner, who left a trail of paper to follow. The Crick Run in England in 1838 was the first recorded instance of an organised cross country competition. The sport gained popularity in British, then American schools in the 19th century and culminated in the creation of the first International Cross Country Championships in 1903. The annual IAAF World Cross Country Championships was inaugurated in 1973 and this remains the highest level of competition for the sport. A number of continental cross country competitions are held, with championships taking place in Africa, Asia, Europe, Oceania, North America and South America. The sport has retained its status at the scholastic level, particularly in the United Kingdom and United States. At the professional level, the foremost competitions come under the banner of the IAAF Cross Country Permit Meetings.

While cross country competitions are no longer held at the Olympics, having featured in the athletics programme from 1912–1924, it has been present as one of the events within the modern pentathlon competition since the 1912 Summer Olympics.

Fell running, trail running and mountain running can all be considered variations on traditional cross country which incorporate significant uphill and/or downhill sections as an additional challenge to the course.

Endurance Training

Endurance training is the act of exercising to increase endurance. The term endurance training generally refers to training the aerobic system as opposed to the anaerobic system. The need for endurance in sports is often predicated as the need of cardiovascular and simple muscular endurance, but the issue of endurance is far more complex. Endurance can be divided into two categories including: general endurance and specific endurance. It can be shown that endurance in sport is closely tied to the execution of skill and technique. A well conditioned athlete can be defined as, the athlete who executes his or her technique consistently and effectively with the least effort.

Endurance training is essential for a variety of endurance sports. A notable example is distance running events (800 meters upwards to marathon and ultra-marathon) with the required degree of endurance training increasing with race distance. Two other popular examples are cycling (particularly road cycling) and competitive swimming. These three endurance sports are combined in triathlon. Other sports for which extensive amounts of endurance training are required include rowing and cross country skiing. Athletes can also undergo endurance training when their sport may not necessarily be an endurance sport in the whole sense but may still demand some endurance. For instance aerobic endurance is necessary (to varying extents) in racket sports, football, rugby, martial arts, basketball and cricket. Endurance exercise tends to be popular with non-athletes for the purpose of increasing general fitness or burning more calories to increase weight loss potential.

Physiological Effects

Long-term endurance training induces many physiological adaptations both centrally and peripherally mediated. Central cardiovascular adaptations include decreased heart rate, increased stroke volume of the heart, increased blood plasma, without any major changes in red blood cell count, which reduces blood viscosity and increased cardiac output as well as total mitochondrial volume in the muscle fibers used in the training (i.e. the thigh muscles in runners will have more mitochondria than the thigh muscles of swimmers). Mitochondria increase in both number and size and there are similar increases in myoglobin and oxidative enzymes. Adaptations of the peripheral include capillarization, that is an increase in the surface area that both the venous and arterial capillaries supply. This also allows for increased heat dissipation during strenuous exercise. The muscles heighten their glycogen and fat storing capabilities in endurance athletes in order to increase the length in time in which they can perform work. Endurance training primarily work the slow twitch (type 1) fibers and develop such fibers in their efficiency and resistance to fatigue. Catabolism also improves increasing the athletes capacity to use fat and glycogen stores as an energy source. These metabolic processes are known as glycogenolysis, glycolysis and lipolysis. There is higher efficiency in oxygen transport and distribution. In recent years it has been recognized that oxidative enzymes such as succinate dehydrogenase (SDH) that enable mitochondria to break down nutrients to form ATP increase by 2.5 times in well trained endurance athletes In addition to SDH, myoglobin increases by 75-80% in well trained endurance athletes.

Risks of Excessive Endurance Training

The potential for negative health effects from long-term, high-volume endurance training have begun to emerge in the scientific literature in recent years. The known risks are primarily associated with training for and participation in extreme endurance events, and affect the cardiovascular system through adverse structural remodeling of the heart and the associated arteries, with heart-rhythm abnormalities perhaps being the most common resulting symptom. Endurance exercise can also reduce testosterone levels.

Methods and Training Plans

Common methods for training include periodization, intervals, hard easy, long slow distance, and in recent years high-intensity interval training. The periodization method is very common and was accredited to Tudor Bompa and consists of blocks of time, generally 4–12 weeks each. The blocks are called preparation, base, build and race. The goal of a structured training program with periodization is to bring the athlete into peak fitness at the time of a big race or event. Preparation as the name suggests lays the groundwork for heavier work to follow. For a runner contemplating a competitive marathon the preparation phase might consist of easier runs of 1–4 miles 3-4 times per week and including 2–3 days of core strengthening. In the base, phase the athlete now works on building cardiovascular endurance by having several long runs staying in heart rate zone 1-2 every week and each week adding slightly more mileage (using 10% rule for safely increasing the mileage). Core strengthening is continued in the base period. Once the base phase is complete and the athlete has sufficient endurance, the build period is needed to give the athlete the ability to hold a faster pace for the race duration. The build phase is where duration of runs is traded for intensity or heart rate zones 3-5. An easy method to obtain intensity is interval training and interval training starts to happen in the build phase. Through interval training during the build phase the athlete can achieve higher lactate threshold and in some athletes VO2 max is increased. Because interval training is demanding on the body, a professional coach should be consulted. In the very least the athlete should do a warm up and active stretching before the interval session and static stretch or yoga after hard interval sessions. It is also advisable to have days of rest or easy workouts the day after interval sessions. Finally the race phase of the periodization approach is where the duration of the workouts decreases but intense workouts remain so as to keep the high lactate threshold that was gained in the build phase. In Ironman training, the race phase is where a long "taper" occurs of up to 4 weeks for highly trained Ironman racers. A final phase is designated transition and is a period of time, where the body is allowed to recover from the hard race effort and some maintenance endurance training is performed so the high fitness level attained in the previous periods will not be lost.

Traditionally, strength training (the performance of exercises with resistance or added weight) was not deemed appropriate for endurance athletes due to potential interference in the adaptive response to the endurance elements of an athlete's training plan. There were also misconceptions regarding the addition of excess body mass through muscle hypertrophy (growth) associated with strength training, which could negatively effect endurance performance by increasing the amount of work required to be completed by the athlete. However, more recent and comprehensive research has proved that short-term (8 weeks) strength training in addition to endurance training is beneficial for endurance performance, particularly long-distance running.

Devices to Assess Endurance Fitness

The heart rate monitor is one of the relatively easy methods to assess fitness in endurance athletes. By comparing heart rate over time fitness gains can be observed when the heart rate decreases for running or cycling at a given speed. In cycling the effect of wind on the cyclists speed is difficult to subtract out and so many cyclists now use power meters built into their bicycles. The power meter allows the athlete to actually measure power output over a set duration or course and allows direct comparison of fitness progression. In the 2008 Olympics, Michael Phelps was aided by repeated lactate threshold measurement. This allowed his coaches to fine tune his training program so that he could recover between swim events that were sometimes several minutes apart. Much similar to blood glucose for diabetes, lower priced lactate measurement devices are now available but in general the lactate measurement approach is still the domain of the professional coach and elite athlete.

Jogging

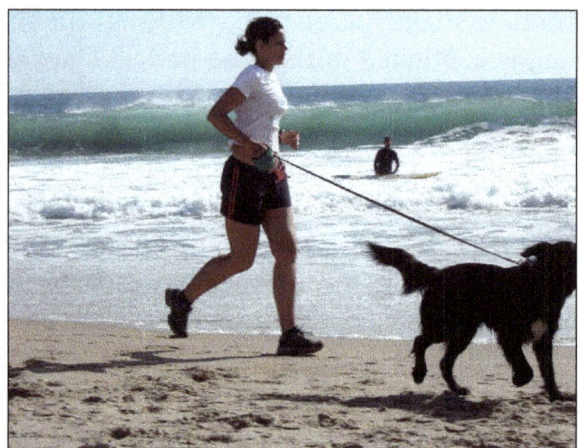

Woman jogging with a dog on Carcavelos Beach.

Jogging is a form of trotting or running at a slow or leisurely pace. The main intention is to increase physical fitness with less stress on the body than from faster running but more than walking, or to maintain a steady speed for longer periods of time. Performed over long distances, it is a form of aerobic endurance training.

Jogging is running at a gentle pace, its definition, as compared with running, is not standard. One definition describes jogging as running slower than 6 miles per hour (10 km/h). Running is sometimes defined as requiring a moment of no contact to the ground, whereas jogging often sustains the contact.

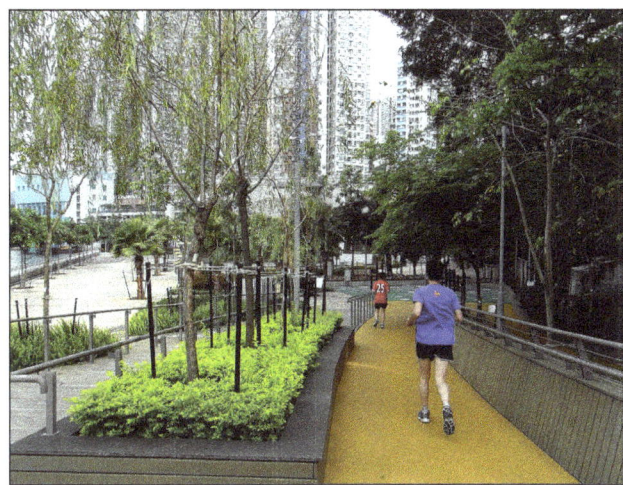
Jogging track in Hong Kong.

Jogging is also distinguished from running by having a wider lateral spacing of foot strikes, creating side-to-side movement that likely adds stability at slower speeds or when coordination is lacking.

Exercise

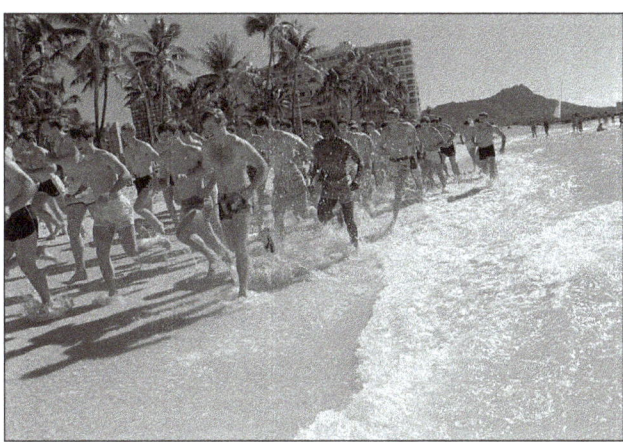
Members of the United States Air Force Academy American football team jog on Waikiki beach, Hawaii.

Jogging may also be used as a warm up or cool down for runners, preceding or following a workout or race. It is often used by serious runners as a means of active recovery during interval training. For example, a runner who completes a fast 400 metre repetition at a sub-5-minute mile pace (3 minute km) may drop to an 8-minute mile jogging pace (5 minute km) for a recovery lap.

Jogging can be used as a method to increase endurance or to provide a means of cardiovascular exercise but with less stress on joints or demand on the circulatory system.

Benefits

Jogging is effective in increasing human lifespan, and decreasing the effects of aging, with benefits for the cardiovascular system. Jogging is useful for fighting obesity and staying healthy.

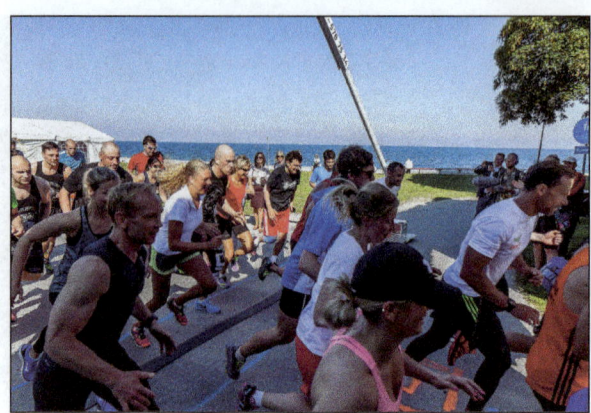
Säpojoggen jogging event in Sweden.

The National Cancer Institute has performed studies that suggest jogging and other types of aerobic exercise can reduce the risk of lung, colon, breast and prostate cancers, among others. It is suggested by the American Cancer Society that jogging for at least 30 minutes five days a week can help in cancer prevention.

While jogging on a treadmill will provide health benefits such as cancer prevention, and aid in weight loss, a study published in BMC Public Health reports that jogging outdoors can have the additional benefits of increased energy and concentration. Jogging outdoors is a better way to improve energy levels and advance mood than using a treadmill at the gym.

Jogging also prevents muscle and bone damage that often occurs with age, improves heart performance and blood circulation and assists in preserving a balanced weight gain.

"Light" and "moderate" jogging were associated with reduced mortality compared to both non-jogging and "strenuous" jogging. The optimal amount per week was 1 to 2.4 hours, the optimal frequency was less than or equal to 3 times per week and the optimal speed was "slow" or "average".

Walking

People often consider walking more of a recreation than a sport, believing it less beneficial to your health compared to "real exercise." What these people seem to forget is that exercise is not measured solely in sweat. If included as part of a routine fitness plan, walking can get your heart pumping, muscles working, and fat burning—all of the things that a real workout is meant to achieve.

Cardiovascular Benefits

Walking at a brisk pace raises your heart rate to a moderate intensity level beneficial to your cardiovascular health. As a reference point, a brisk pace is one to where you are able to talk but won't have the lung capacity to sing.

If you take your pulse in the moderate intensity zone, it should be between 50 percent and 70 percent of your maximum heart rate (MHR). Your MHR can be roughly estimated by subtracting your age from 220.

In order to achieve tangible benefits, aim for a minimum of 30 minutes of moderate-intensity exercise per day, five days a week. You don't have to do it all at once; you can break it into sessions of no less than 10 minutes each.

20-minute brisk walking workout:

- Start at an easy pace for one to three minutes to warm up.

- Increase to 50 to 70 percent of your MHR for 20 minutes.

- To cool down, slow to an easy pace for one to three minutes.

Aerobic Fitness

By walking at a vigorous pace, you can improve your aerobic fitness. Doing so moves your heart rate into a moderate-high intensity zone of 70 percent to 80 percent of your MHR. At this pace, you will be able to speak but not in full sentences.

By doing this for 30 minutes per day, at least three to four days a week, you can increase your lung capacity and improve the transfer of oxygen to the bloodstream.

You can achieve this pace by not only walking faster but by increasing the incline on your treadmill, walking up hills, or combining walking with short jogging intervals.

Try this aerobic walking workout:

- Start at an easy pace for five minutes.

- Increase to 70 to 80 percent of your MHR for 30 to 50 minutes.

- Cool down by walking an easy pace for five minutes.

Weight Control

One of the benefits of routine walking is that it can help you control your weight or even shed a few pounds when combined a reduced-calorie diet.

While 45 minutes of brisk walking can encourage your body to burn stored fat, it can only do so if you don't replace those fats in your diet. To the end, it is important to speak with your doctor or nutritionist to ensure you are burning more calories than you consume and that you do so safely.

Try this fat-burning walking workout:

- Start at an easy to moderate pace for 10 minutes.

- Increase to 60 to 70 percent of your MHR for 30 to 60 minutes.

- Cool down with five to 10 minutes at an easy pace.

Muscles and Joints

Walking is beneficial even if you are unable to do so at a brisk pace. Walking at an easy pace works your muscles and joints, improving your flexibility and strength even when you are not being aerobically challenged.

Walking regularly is especially helpful if you are overweight or living with arthritis. By walking at a slower pace, you minimize the stress on your knees, ankles, hips, and lower back.

While it doesn't have the cardiovascular benefits of brisk walking, low-intensity walking can slow joint deterioration and improve your mood and energy levels if done consistently. There is also evidence it can improve your metabolic health.

Just two minutes of low-intensity walking done every 20 minutes improved blood sugar control in obese people compared to those who simply sat or stood still.

The same benefits can be extended to office workers who spend much of their day behind a desk. Getting up and walking for a few minutes can translate the better health irrespective of your age or health status.

If you are addicted to your fitness tracker and make an effort to reach 10,000 steps per day, you are certainly on the right track to achieving good health. But don't mistake the number of steps for the quality of a workout. Clearly, 10,000 steps done a low-intensity is unlikely to deliver the same health benefits as 5,000 done at a strenuous pace.

When starting a walking program, be clear about your goals and what you need to do to achieve them. Higher quality trackers, like Fitbit, are able to analyze your steps and tell you how many have been done at an aerobic pace. If you want to ensure you are getting "real exercise," focus on that latter figure and not just the step count.

Techniques for Effective Exercise Walking

There are several stretches and techniques that will improve the benefits of exercise walking, as well as help prevent injury.

Stretching before Walking

Prior to exercise walking, gentle stretching should be done to prepare the joints and muscles for the increased range of motion needed. It is important to take an easy five minute walk to warm up the muscles before stretching so they're not completely cold when stretching.

Discuss with a healthcare practitioner the best way to do stretches, and be sure to include the neck, arms, hips, upper and lower leg muscles (including the hamstring muscles in the back of the thigh), and ankles.

Techniques for Exercise Walking

Using the following techniques will help improve the benefits of walking:

- Walk briskly, but as a general rule maintain enough breath to be able to carry on a conversation.

- Start out with a 5 minute walk and work up to walking for at least 30 minutes (roughly 2 miles) at least 3 to 4 times a week.

- Maintain good form while walking to get the optimum aerobic benefit with each step and help protect the back and avoid injury. These elements of form should be followed:

  ○ Head and shoulders: Keep the head up and centered between the shoulders, with eyes focused straight ahead at the horizon. Keep the shoulders relaxed but straight - avoid slouching forward.

  ○ Abdominal muscles: It is important to actively use the abdominal muscles to help support the trunk of the body and the spine. To do this, keep the stomach pulled in slightly and stand fully upright. Avoid leaning forward as you walk.

  ○ Hips: The majority of the forward motion should start with the hips. Each stride should feel natural - not too long or too short. Most people make the mistake of trying to take too long of stride.

Cross-training

Cross training is typically defined as an exercise regimen that uses several modes of training to develop a specific component of fitness.

What are the Benefits of Cross Training?

Here are few of the numerous documented benefits cross training has to offer:

- Reduced risk of injury: By spreading the cumulative level of orthopedic stress over additional muscles and joints, individuals are able to exercise more frequently and for longer durations without excessively overloading particularly vulnerable areas of the body (e.g., knees, hips, back, shoulders, elbows and feet). People who are particularly prone to lower-leg problems from running long distances should consider incorporating low-impact activities such as elliptical training, cycling and swimming into their regimens. It should be noted, however, that competitive cross-trainers can experience certain overuse injuries due to inadequate muscle rest, an unbalanced workout schedule, or both.

- Enhanced weight loss: Individuals who want to lose weight and body fat should engage in an exercise program that enables them to safely burn a significant number of calories. Research has shown that such a goal, in most instances, is best accomplished when individuals exercise for relatively long durations (i.e., more than 30 minutes) at a moderate level of intensity (i.e., 60 percent to 85 percent of maximal heart rate). Overweight individuals can effectively achieve a reduction in body weight and fat stores by combining two or more physical activities in a cross-training regimen. They can, for example, exercise on an elliptical trainer for 20 to 30 minutes and then cycle for an additional 20 to 30 minutes.

- Improved total fitness: Cross training can include activities that develop muscular fitness, as well as aerobic conditioning. While an individual's muscular fitness gains will typically be less than if he or she participated only in strength training, the added benefits of improving muscular strength and endurance can pay substantial dividends. For example, research has shown that resistance training can help individuals prevent injury, control body weight and improve functional capacity.

- Enhanced exercise adherence: Research on exercise adherence indicates that many individuals drop out of exercise programs because they become bored or injured. Cross training is a safe and relatively easy way to add variety to an exercise program. In the process, it can play a positive role in promoting long-term exercise adherence by reducing the incidence of injury and eliminating or diminishing the potential for boredom.

The essential fundamentals of cross training are the same whether you are exercising for improved health and fitness or for competition. Try varying your exercise program from workout to workout by engaging in different types of activities, or simply add a new form of exercise (e.g., resistance training, Pilates, a boot-camp class) to your existing workout routine.

One of the easiest ways to incorporate cross training is to alternate between activities (e.g., run one day, stair climb the next, cycle the next). You can also alternate activities within a single workout (e.g., walk on a treadmill for 10 minutes, exercise on an elliptical trainer for 10 minutes and cycle for 10 minutes, for a total of 30 minutes of exercise).

Burpee

The burpee, or squat thrust, is a full body exercise used in strength training and as an aerobic exercise. The basic movement is performed in four steps and known as a "four-count burpee":

- Begin in a standing position.
- Move into a squat position with your hands on the ground.
- Kick your feet back into a plank position, while keeping your arms extended.
- Immediately return your feet into squat position.
- Stand up from the squat position.

Progression

The way to perform a burpee as originally intended has progressed since the 1930s. The up phase of the burpee used to be with the feet landing between the hands while still grounded, which creates unnecessary pressure on the lower back. It's now more common to land the feet on the outside of the hands.

Confusion

The burpee is sometimes confused with a sprawl. A sprawl is similar to the burpee with the main difference being that the hips are thrust towards the ground in the plank position.

Variants

Box-jump burpee: The athlete jumps onto a box, rather than straight up and down.

Burpee broad jump: A burpee followed by a stationary two footed distance jump.

Burpee push up (also known as a "bastardo"): The athlete performs one push-up after assuming the extended plank position.

CrossFit burpee: The athlete performs a standard four count burpee with the addition of a tricep push up at the bottom, where the chest and thighs touch the floor, and jump at the top of the standing position with hands above the head.

CrossFit speed burpee: The athlete drops to the ground with the chest and thighs touching the floor, creating a hollow back through hip extension, rolling onto the knees getting up, and perform a jump with hands above the head. This version is all about efficiency, high reps.

Dumbbell burpee: The athlete holds a pair of dumbbells while performing the exercise.

Eight-count push up or Double burpee: The athlete performs two push-ups after assuming the plank position. This cancels the drive from landing after the jump and makes the next jump harder. Each part of the burpee might be repeated to make it even harder.

Hindu push up burpee: Instead of a regular push up, do a Hindu push up.

Jump-over burpee: The athlete jumps over an obstacle between burpees.

Jump up burpee: The athlete jumps straight up as high as possible at the end of the movement, before beginning the next burpee.

Knee push-up burpee: The athlete bends their knees and rests them on the ground before performing the push up.

Long-jump burpee: The athlete jumps forward, not upward.

Muscle-up burpee: Combine a muscle-up (a variation of a pull-up) with the jump or do a muscle-up instead of the jump.

One-armed burpee: The athlete uses only one arm for the whole exercise including the pushup.

One leg burpee: The athlete stands on one leg, bends at the waist and puts hands on ground so they are aligned with shoulders. Next jump back with the standing leg to plank position. Jump forward with the one leg that was extended, and do a one-leg jump. Repeat on opposite side.

Parkour burpee: Following one burpee on the ground, the athlete jumps upon a table and performs the second burpee on the table, then jumps back to the initial position.

Pull-up burpee: Combine a pull-up with the jump or do a pull-up instead of the jump.

Side burpee: The athlete bends at waist and places hand shoulder-width apart to the side of right or left foot. Jump both legs out to side and land on the outer and inner sides of your feet. Jump back in, jump up, and repeat on opposite side.

Squat thrust: Same as a four-count burpee.

Tuck-jump burpee: The athlete pulls their knees to their chest (tucks) at the peak of the jump.

Swimming

Water is Calming

Water has long been a symbol of renewal and clarity and there's research to back this up. Studies suggest being around the element has a powerful effect on the brain.

Spending time near water can be similar to meditation, in that it gives the brain a break from the constant overstimulation people often experience in modern life. You can reap these cognitive benefits by going for a swim and getting some exercise in the process. You could also give floating therapy a try.

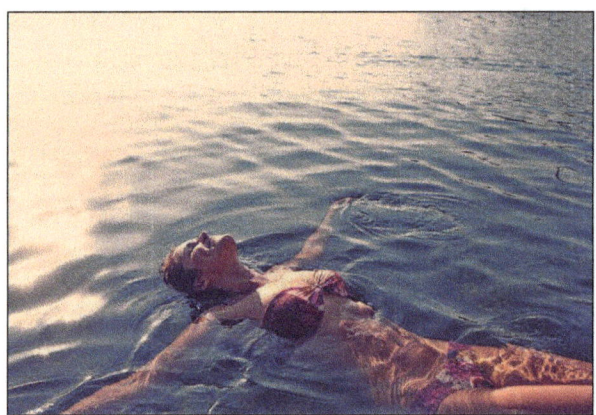

Swimming is Low Impact

Unlike jogging or plyometric training, swimming is a way to fit cardio into your workout routine without putting stress on your bones, joints and muscles. This is a plus for swimmers of all ages and body types, but it's particularly beneficial for seniors and people with arthritis. It's one of the best ways to stay active while taking care of all parts of your body.

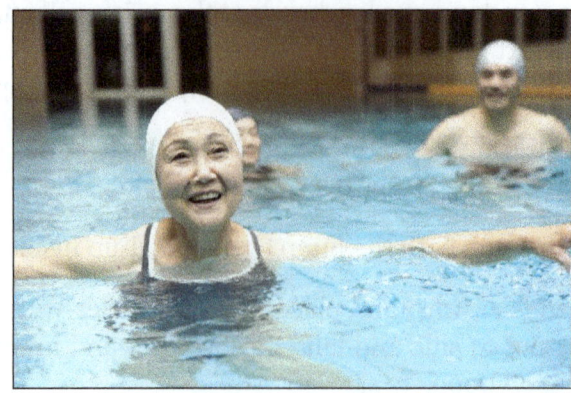

It can Bring you Closer to Nature

If you're lucky enough to live near the ocean or a lake, opting to swim in a natural body of water could be even better for your health. Studies show that spending time in nature can improve your mental and physical well-being by helping you maintain a healthy weight, reducing stress and boosting your mood.

Plus, becoming a stronger swimmer might open doors to other water-based activities like snorkeling or surfing. A lifelong love of all things aquatic starts with dipping your toes in the shallow end.

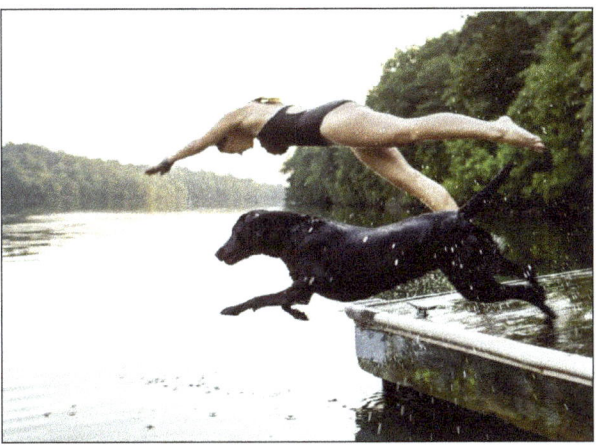

Swimming Builds Strength and Cardio Abilities Simultaneously

Though it's a low-impact workout, swimming produces high-power results. It is typically considered an aerobic exercise, but exercising in water also provides moderate resistance. This can in turn build strength.

Building and maintaining muscle, especially as you grow older, is essential for a healthy body and a long life. Resistance training also improves balance, sleep and bone health. Talk about a total-body workout.

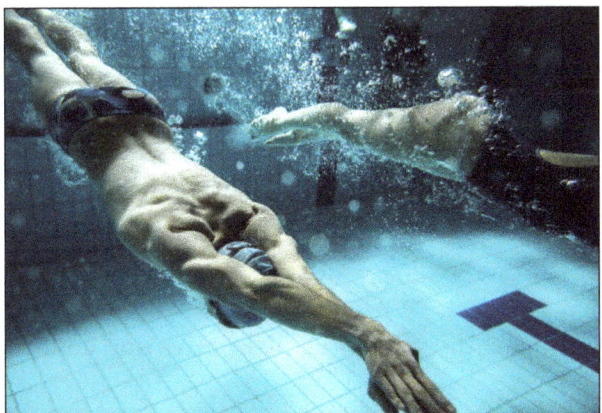

It could help Maintain Healthy Lungs

Some research suggests there's a link between swimmers and a better lung capacity.

With healthy lungs, the body can process oxygen more proficiently this means you won't feel winded or out of breath as easily. Stronger lungs might also help you ward off illness. A 2007 study found a link between reduced lung capacity and cardiovascular disease.

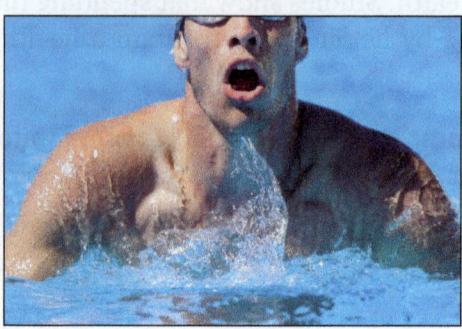

Essentially, swimming reigns supreme for maintaining a healthy body and mind.

Benefits of Swimming

Swimming is a great workout because you need to move your whole body against the resistance of the water.

Swimming is a good all-round activity because it:

- Keeps your heart rate up but takes some of the impact stress off your body.

- Builds endurance, muscle strength and cardiovascular fitness.

- Helps maintain a healthy weight, healthy heart and lungs.

- Tones muscles and builds strength.

- Provides an all-over body workout, as nearly all of your muscles are used during swimming.

Other Benefits of Swimming

Swimming has many other benefits including:

- Being a relaxing and peaceful form of exercise.

- Alleviating stress.

- Improving coordination, balance and posture.

- Improving flexibility.

- Providing good low-impact therapy for some injuries and conditions.

- Providing a pleasant way to cool down on a hot day.

- Being available in many places – you can swim in swimming pools, beaches, lakes, dams and rivers. Make sure that the environment you choose to swim in is safe.

References

- Aerobic-exercise: sciencedaily.com, Retrieved 26 July, 2019

- Aerobic-respiration: biologydictionary.net, Retrieved 21 May, 2019

- Li xb, gu jd, zhou qh (january 2015). "review of aerobic glycolysis and its key enzymes - new targets for lung cancer therapy". Thoracic cancer. 6 (1): 17–24. Doi:10.1111/1759-7714.12148. Pmc 4448463. Pmid 26273330

- What-are-other-options-for-aerobic-exercise, aerobic-exercise: emedicinehealth.com, Retrieved 8 January, 2019

- Piotrowska-calka, e.e. (2010). "effects of a 24-week deep water aerobic training program on cardiovascular fitness". Biology of sport. Retrieved 2013-11-10

- Spinning, health-fitness: edinformatics.com, Retrieved 13 May, 2019

- "Father of aerobics" kenneth cooper, md, mph to receive healthy cup award from harvard school of public health". News. 2008-04-16. Retrieved 2018-10-08

- Aerobic-exercise-the-health-benefits, sports-fitness: mydr.com.au, Retrieved 25 February, 2019

- Swimming-health-benefits, healthyliving, health: gov.au, Retrieved 16 January, 2019

4
Anaerobic Exercise

A type of physical exercise which is used by athletes in non-endurance sports for improvement in strength, speed and power is referred to as anaerobic exercise. A few of such exercises are strength training, stretching and sprinting. This chapter has been carefully written to provide an easy understanding of these anaerobic exercises.

Anaerobic exercise means you are working at such high intensity that your cardiovascular system can't deliver oxygen to your muscles fast enough . That doesn't sound like a desirable outcome, but this type of activity can improve both your endurance and muscle strength. And because muscles need oxygen to continue working, anaerobic exercises can only last for short periods, allowing you to cut your total workout time.

If you've ever gotten completely breathless during a workout, or made it to 90 percent to 100 percent of your maximum heart rate, you know what anaerobic exercise feels like. Both cardio and strength training activities can be anaerobic. The biggest difference between aerobic ("with oxygen") and anaerobic exercise is the intensity at which you are working.

Benefits of Anaerobic Exercise

While anaerobic exercise used to be something that mainly athletes did to increase performance, everyday exercisers can also benefit from this type of training. When you train at high levels of intensity, you increase your anaerobic threshold. That means you can work harder for longer periods of time, all while burning more calories.

Other benefits include:

- Endurance: Do some anaerobic training and your other workouts will get easier.

- Improved VO_2 max: Your body learns how to use more oxygen, which it converts into energy to allow you to exercise longer.

- Stronger muscles: Instead of producing energy from oxygen (as it does during aerobic workouts), your body uses energy stores in the muscles during anaerobic exercise. That means it helps maintain and improve muscle mass.

- Stronger bones: Some anaerobic exercise (such as intense resistance training) can improve bone density and strength. This, in turn, reduces the risk of osteoporosis.

- Fat loss: One study found that high-intensity intermittent exercise (that is, interval training) can be more effective than aerobic workouts at helping exercisers burn fat.

- Improved mood: Just like aerobic exercise, anaerobic training has been shown to decrease feelings of depression, tension, and anger.

Considerations

This is a very challenging way of exercising, so don't start here if you're a beginner. Going too hard and fast could put you at risk for injury and discomfort, so start with aerobic interval training offered by a beginner interval workout.

Once you do work up to incorporating some anaerobic exercise into your workouts, remember that you'll need full recovery afterward.

You should only do this type of exercise two to three times a week with rest days in between.

Adding Anaerobic Exercise to your Workouts

Anaerobic activities can be cardio exercises or dynamic strength training options such as:

- Sprints

- Fartlek training

- High-intensity interval training (HIIT)

- Tabata training

- Certain types of kettlebell training

- Powerlifting

- Plyometric training

- Metabolic conditioning

You can try these or similar options, or add bursts of very high-intensity cardio to a regular steady-state workout. For example, if you're running on a treadmill, hop off every five minutes and do 30 to 60 seconds of intense cardio exercises like these:

- Plyo jacks

- Plyo lunges

- Froggy jumps

- Squat jumps

Aerobic vs. Anaerobic Exercise

It's important to remember that, while the names sound similar, there is a difference between aerobic and anaerobic exercise. The key difference is that they use different energy systems. Aerobic exercise uses energy stored in the body from fats, carbs, and proteins, along with oxygen from breathing, to make energy available to the muscles. Anaerobic exercise, on the other hand, uses energy stored in the muscles. Aerobic exercises burn calories during the activity only, while anaerobic exercise burns calories even when the body is at rest. And while aerobic exercises tend to develop stamina, anaerobic exercises focus on developing force.

Benefits of Anaerobic Exercise

Anaerobic exercise is beneficial for the body and promotes good health by building muscle, burning fats, strengthening bones, and maintaining muscle mass, which is particularly important as you age.

Builds Muscle

One of the most popular anaerobic exercise benefits is that it helps build lean muscle mass and improve endurance and fitness levels. Increased lean muscle mass due to exercise boosts the metabolism and helps combat fatigue. It also helps reduce body fat, which is a key factor for people trying to achieve weight loss goals.

Improves Mood

Exercising has been shown to reduce symptoms of anxiety and depression. It also relieves stress, helps you sleep better, improves your memory, and boosts your overall mood. Engaging in exercise releases endorphins — chemicals released in the brain that trigger a positive feeling, similar to that of morphine — that energize your spirits and make you feel good. Finally, anaerobic exercise can also serve as a distraction, helping you to find a calm and relaxing time to break out of the cycle of negative feelings that feed depression.

Increases Endurance

Anaerobic exercise helps build endurance and fitness levels. In fact, many lower body strength training exercises are designed to increase stamina and endurance.

Lowers Blood Sugar

The body turns the food you eat into sugar. Food that remains unused is either burned immediately, stored as fat in the body, or stored as glycogen in the muscles. Regular anaerobic exercise helps regulate insulin by burning the stored glycogen in order to help your body stay healthy. This helps you avoid spikes in blood sugar levels.

Raises VO2 Max

VO2 max is the greatest quantity of oxygen the body is capable of consuming during exercise. The average VO2 max for untrained, healthy males is about 35–40 mL/(kg·min), and for healthy females about 27–31 mL/(kg·min). Regular anaerobic exercise helps increase these numbers. This is significant because it allows the body more oxygen to perform swift bursts of activity in your daily life, and also helps improve endurance for other activities, like aerobic activity.

Increases Metabolism

High-intensity anaerobic exercise makes the muscles in the body hungry. After an intense workout, your metabolism functions at a higher rate of speed for several hours. Repeated exercise and workout build larger muscles, which raise your resting metabolic rate and result in the body burning more calories — even in your sleep.

Boosts Energy

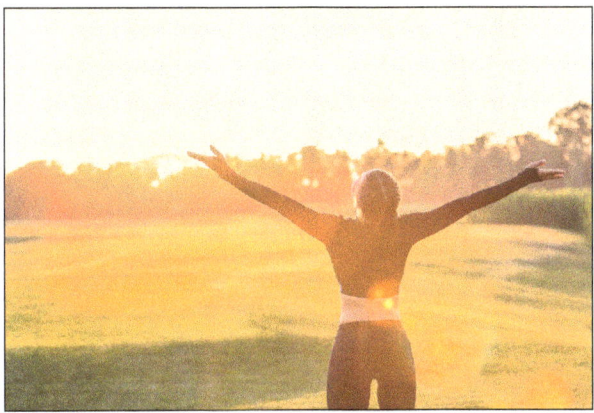

Your body depends on the glycogen stored in your muscles for energy. Regular anaerobic exercise boosts and enhances your body's tendency to store glycogen, providing you with more energy when you need it.

Protects Joints

Regular anaerobic exercise increases muscle strength, and this additional muscle mass and strength translates to joint protection in the body. The result? You're less likely to get injured.

Improves Bone Strength and Density

Anaerobic exercises increase bone density, which helps prevent osteoporosis (bone loss) that happens naturally as the body ages.

Promotes Fat Loss

Anaerobic exercise like high-intensity intermittent training (HIIT) helps you burn fat more quickly than with aerobic exercise. It also helps fade away the appearance of cellulite by plumping up the collagen in your skin.

Reduces the Risk of Disease

Anaerobic workouts are best for burning calories and fighting fat — and maintaining a healthy weight is key to good overall health and well being. Anaerobic training also improves overall cardiopulmonary health. Strengthened bone density attained by high-intensity anaerobic training (like push-ups and bodyweight squats) reduces the risk of diseases like diabetes, heart disease, and rheumatoid arthritis (RA).

Strength Training

Strength training is a type of physical exercise specializing in the use of resistance to induce muscular contraction, which builds the strength, anaerobic endurance, size of skeletal muscles and bone density.

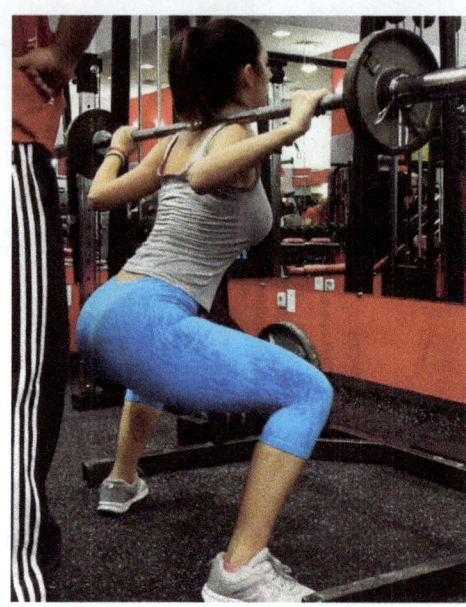

When properly performed, strength training can provide significant functional benefits and improvement in overall health and well-being, including increased bone, muscle, tendon, and ligament strength and toughness, improved joint function, reduced potential for injury, increased bone density, increased metabolism, increased fitness and improved cardiac function. Training commonly uses the technique of progressively increasing the force output of the muscle through incremental weight increases and uses a variety of exercises and types of equipment to target specific muscle groups. Strength training is primarily an anaerobic activity, although some proponents have adapted it to provide the benefits of aerobic exercise through circuit training.

Strength training is typically associated with the production of lactate, which is a limiting factor of exercise performance. Regular endurance exercise leads to adaptations in skeletal muscle which can prevent lactate levels from rising during strength training. This is mediated via activation of PGC-1alpha which alter the LDH (lactate dehydrogenase) isoenzyme complex composition and decreases the activity of the lactate generating enzyme LDHA, while increasing the activity of the lactate metabolizing enzyme LDHB.

Sports where strength training is central are bodybuilding, weightlifting, powerlifting, strongman, Highland games, shot put, discus throw, and javelin throw. Many other sports use strength training as part of their training regimen, notably tennis, American football, wrestling, track and field, rowing, lacrosse, basketball, pole dancing, hockey, professional wrestling, rugby union, rugby league, and soccer. Strength training for other sports and physical activities is becoming increasingly popular.

Uses

The benefits of strength training include greater muscular strength, improved muscle tone and appearance, increased endurance and enhanced bone density.

Increased Physical Attractiveness

Many people take up strength training to improve their physical attractiveness. There is evidence that a body type consisting of broad shoulders and a narrow waist, attainable through strength training, is the most physically attractive male attribute according to women participating in the research. Most men can develop substantial muscles; most women lack the testosterone to do it, but they can develop a firm, "toned" physique, and they can increase their strength by the same proportion as that achieved by men (but usually from a significantly lower starting point). An individual's genetic make-up dictates the response to weight training stimuli to a significant extent. Training can not exceed a muscle's intrinsic genetically determined qualities, though polymorphic expression does occur e.g., Myosin heavy chains.

Studies also show that people are able to tell the strength of men based on photos of their bodies and faces, and that physical appearance indicates cues of strengths that are often linked to a man's physical formidability and, therefore, his attractiveness. This is aligned with studies that reveal those who undergo strength training attain more self-esteem and body cathexis when compared to individuals who do not undergo training or exercise. In addition, people who undergo strength training tend to have a more favorable body image even than those who also engage in regular physical activities such as walking and running. More women are also increasingly revealed to be dissatisfied with their body today than those surveyed in 1984 and they often turn to exercise such as strength training to improve their body shape.

Workouts elevate metabolism for up to 14 hours following 45-minutes of vigorous exercise.

Increased General Physical Health

Strength training also provides functional benefits. Stronger muscles improve posture, provide better support for joints, and reduce the risk of injury from everyday activities. Older people who take up weight training can prevent some of the loss of muscle tissue that normally accompanies aging—and even regain some functional strength—and by doing so become less frail. They may be able to avoid some types of physical disability. Weight-bearing exercise also helps to prevent osteoporosis and to improve bone strength in those with osteoporosis. The benefits of weight training for older people have been confirmed by studies of people who began engaging in it even in their 80s and 90s.

Though strength training can stimulate the cardiovascular system, many exercise physiologists, based on their observation of maximal oxygen uptake, argue that aerobics training is a better cardiovascular stimulus. Central catheter monitoring during resistance training reveals increased cardiac output, suggesting that strength training shows potential for cardiovascular exercise. However, a 2007 meta-analysis found that, though aerobic training is an effective therapy for heart failure patients, combined aerobic and strength training is ineffective.

Strength training may be important to metabolic and cardiovascular health. Recent evidence suggests that resistance training may reduce metabolic and cardiovascular disease risk. Overweight individuals with high strength fitness exhibit metabolic/cardiovascular risk profiles similar to normal-weight, fit individuals rather than overweight unfit individuals.

For Rehabilitation or to Address an Impairment

For many people in rehabilitation or with an acquired disability, such as following stroke or orthopaedic surgery, strength training for weak muscles is a key factor to optimise recovery. For people with such a health condition, their strength training is likely to need to be designed by an appropriate health professional, such as a physiotherapist or an occupational therapist.

Increased Sports Performance

Stronger muscles improve performance in a variety of sports. Sport-specific training routines are used by many competitors. These often specify that the speed of muscle contraction during weight training should be the same as that of the particular sport.

Technique

The basic principles of strength training involve a manipulation of the number of repetitions, sets, tempo, exercises and force to cause desired changes in strength, endurance or size by overloading of a group of muscles. The specific combinations of reps, sets, exercises, resistance and force depend on the purpose of the individual performing the exercise: to gain size and strength multiple (4+) sets with fewer reps must be performed using more force. A wide spectrum of regimens can be adopted to achieve different results, but the classic formula recommended by the American College of Sports Medicine reads as follows:

- 8 to 12 repetitions of a resistance training exercise for each major muscle group at an intensity of 40% to 80% of a one-repetition max (RM) depending on the training level of the participant.

- Two to three minutes of rest is recommended between exercise sets to allow for proper recovery.

- Two to four sets are recommended for each muscle group.

Typically, failure to use good form during a training set can result in injury or an inability to meet training goals. When the desired muscle group is not challenged sufficiently, the threshold of overload is never reached and the muscle does not gain in strength. There are cases when cheating is beneficial, as is the case where weaker groups become the weak link in the chain and the target muscles are never fully exercised as a result.

Realization of Training Goals

For developing endurance, gradual increases in volume and gradual decreases in intensity is the most effective program. Sets of thirteen to twenty repetitions develop anaerobic endurance, with some increases to muscle size and limited impact on strength.

It has been shown that for beginners, multiple-set training offers minimal benefits over single-set training with respect to either strength gain or muscle mass increase, but for the experienced athlete multiple-set systems are required for optimal progress. However, one study shows that for leg muscles, three sets are more effective than one set.

Beginning weight-trainers are in the process of training the neurological aspects of strength, the ability of the brain to generate a rate of neuronal action potentials that will produce a muscular contraction that is close to the maximum of the muscle's potential. Table reproduced from Siff, 2003:

Variable	Training goal			
	Strength	Power	Hypertrophy	Endurance
Load (% of 1RM)	90–80	60–45	80–60	60–40
Reps per set	1–5	1–5	6–12	13–60
Sets per exercise	4–7	3–5	4–8	2–4
Rest between sets (mins)	2–6	2–6	2–3	1–2
Duration (seconds per set)	5–10	4–8	20–60	80–150
Speed per rep (% of max)	60–100	90–100	60–90	60–80
Training sessions per week	3–6	3–6	5–7	8–14

Weights for each exercise should be chosen so that the desired number of repetitions can just be achieved.

Progressive Overload

The basic method of weight training uses the principle of progressive overload, in which the muscles are overloaded by attempting to lift at least as much weight as they are capable. They respond by growing larger and stronger. This procedure is repeated with progressively heavier weights as the practitioner gains strength and endurance.

However, performing exercises at the absolute limit of one's strength (known as one rep max lifts) is considered too risky for all but the most experienced practitioners. Moreover, most individuals wish to develop a combination of strength, endurance and muscle size. One repetition sets are not well suited to these aims. Practitioners therefore lift lighter (sub-maximal) weights, with more repetitions, to fatigue the muscle and all fibres within that muscle as required by the progressive overload principle.

Commonly, each exercise is continued to the point of momentary muscular failure. Contrary to widespread belief, this is not the point at which the individual thinks they cannot complete any more repetitions, but rather the first repetition that fails due to inadequate muscular strength. Training to failure is a controversial topic with some advocating training to failure on all sets while others believe that this will lead to overtraining, and suggest training to failure only on the last set of an exercise. Some practitioners recommend finishing a set of repetitions just before reaching a personal maximum at a given time. Adrenaline and other hormones may promote additional intensity by stimulating the body to lift additional weight (as well as the neuro-muscular stimulations that happen when in "fight-or-flight" mode, as the body activates more muscle fibres), so getting "psyched up" before a workout can increase the maximum weight lifted.

Weight training can be a very effective form of strength training because exercises can be chosen, and weights precisely adjusted, to safely exhaust each individual muscle group after the specific numbers of sets and repetitions that have been found to be the most effective for the individual. Other strength training exercises lack the flexibility and precision that weights offer.

Split Training

Split training involves working no more than three muscle groups or body parts per day, instead spreading the training of specific body parts throughout a training cycle of several days. It is commonly used by more advanced practitioners due to the logistics involved in training all muscle groups maximally. Training all the muscles in the body individually through their full range of motion in a single day is generally not considered possible due to caloric and time constraints. Split training involves fully exhausting individual muscle groups during a workout, then allowing several days for the muscle to fully recover. Muscles are worked roughly twice per week and allowed roughly 72 hours to recover. Recovery of certain muscle groups is usually achieved on days while training other groups, i.e. a 7-day week can consist of a practitioner training trapezius, side shoulders and upper shoulders to exhaustion on one day, the following day the arms to exhaustion, the day after that the rear, front shoulders and back, the day after that the chest. In this way all mentioned muscle groups are allowed the necessary recovery.

Perhaps the most common form of training split in recent decades is the body-part split (sometimes known as "bodybuilder split" or "bro split"), which became popular due to being used in professional bodybuilding, and is discussed in a number of sources dedicated to physical training, such as Bodybuilding.com, T-Nation, and Muscle & Strength. This kind of split is structured so that the body is divided up in what are considered the major muscle groups, i.e. chest, back, legs, shoulders, and arms (biceps and triceps), each part is then trained to exhaustion once a week on a dedicated day. Optionally, the biceps can be trained along with the back, due to the fact that they are both involved in pulling movements; conversely, the triceps can be trained along with the chest of the shoulders, as all these muscles are involved in pushing movements. Abdominal work can be spread out over multiple sessions or concentrated on just one day.

Despite the popularity of body-part splits, recent evidence suggests that multiple training sessions for the same muscle group over the course of a week are a more effective training strategy. One recent meta-analysis of experimental trials on resistance training found out that, when total training volume is equated, "frequencies of training twice a week promote superior hypertrophic outcomes to once a week".

Intensity, Volume and Frequency

Three important variables of strength training are intensity, volume, and frequency. Intensity refers to the amount of work required to achieve the activity and is proportional to the mass of the weights being lifted. Volume refers to the number of muscles worked, exercises, sets, and reps during a single session. Frequency refers to how many training sessions are performed per week.

These variables are important because they are all mutually conflicting, as the muscle only has so much strength and endurance, and takes time to recover due to microtrauma. Increasing one by any significant amount necessitates the decrease of the other two, e.g. increasing weight means a reduction of reps, and will require more recovery time and therefore fewer workouts per week. Trying to push too much intensity, volume and frequency will result in overtraining, and eventually lead to injury and other health issues such as chronic soreness and general lethargy, illness or even acute trauma such as avulsion fractures. A high-medium-low formula can be used to avoid overtraining, with either intensity, volume, or frequency being high, one of the others being medium, and the other being low. One example of this training strategy can be found in the following chart:

Type	High	Med	Low
Intensity (% of 1RM)	80–100%	40–70%	0–40%
Volume (per muscle)	3+ exercises	2 exercises	1 exercises
Sets	4+ sets	2–3 sets	1 set
Reps	20+ reps	8–15 reps	1–6 reps
Session frequency	4+ p/w	2–3 p/w	1 p/w

A common training strategy is to set the volume and frequency the same each week (e.g. training 3 times per week, with 2 sets of 12 reps each workout), and steadily increase the intensity (weight) on a weekly basis. However, to maximize progress to specific goals, individual programs may require different manipulations, such as decreasing the weight, and increase volume or frequency.

Making program alterations on a daily basis (daily undulating periodization) seems to be more efficient in eliciting strength gains than doing so every 4 weeks (linear periodization), but for beginners there are no differences between different periodization models.

Periodization

There are many complicated definitions for periodization, but the term simply means the division of the overall training program into periods which accomplish different goals.

Periodization is the modulating of volume, intensity, and frequency over time, to both stimulate gains and allow recovery.

In some programs for example; volume is decreased during a training cycle while intensity is increased. In this template, a lifter would begin a training cycle with a higher rep range than they will finish with.

For this example, the lifter has a 1 rep max of 225 lb:

Week	Set 1	Set 2	Set 3	Set 4	Set 5	Volume Lbs.	% Exertion (Last Set)	% of 1 Rep Max- (Last Set)
1	125 lb x 8reps	130 lb x 8reps	135 lb x 8reps	140 lb x 8reps	145 lb x 8reps	5,400	78%	64%
2	135 lb x 7reps	140 lb x 7reps	145 lb x 7reps	150 lb x 7reps	155 lb x 7reps	5,075	81%	69%
3	145 lb x 6reps	150 lb x 6reps	155 lb x 6reps	160 lb x 6reps	165 lb x 6reps	4,650	84%	73%
4	155 lb x 5reps	160 lb x 5reps	165 lb x 5reps	170 lb x 5reps	175 lb x 5reps	4,125	87%	78%

| 5 | 165 lb x 4reps | 170 lb x 4reps | 175 lb x 4reps | 180 lb x 4reps | 185 lb x 4reps | 3,500 | 90% | 82% |
| 6 | 175 lb x 3reps | 180 lb x 3reps | 185 lb x 3reps | 190 lb x 3reps | 195 lb x 3reps | 2,775 | 92% | 87% |

This is an example of periodization where the number of repetitions decreases while the weight increases.

Practice of Weight Training

Methods and Equipment

There are many methods of strength training. Examples include weight training, circuit training, isometric exercise, gymnastics, plyometrics, Parkour, yoga, Pilates, Super Slow.

Strength training may be done with minimal or no equipment, for instance bodyweight exercises. Equipment used for strength training includes barbells and dumbbells, weight machines and other exercise machines, weighted clothing, resistance bands, gymnastics apparatus, Swiss balls, wobble boards, indian clubs, pneumatic exercise equipment, hydraulic exercise equipment.

Exercises for Specific Muscle Groups

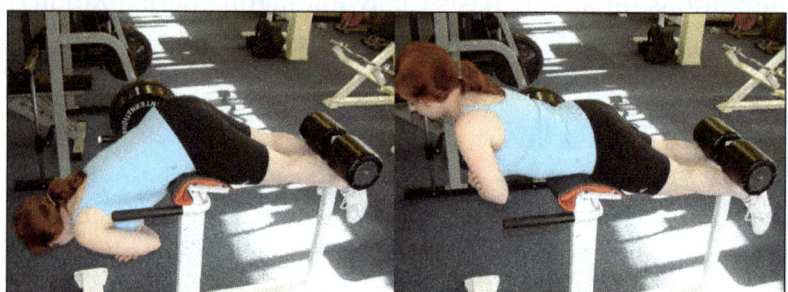

A back extension.

Weight trainers commonly divide the body's individual muscles into ten major muscle groups. These do not include the hip, neck and forearm muscles, which are rarely trained in isolation. The most common exercises for these muscle groups are listed below.

The sequence shown below is one possible way to order the exercises. The large muscles of the lower body are normally trained before the smaller muscles of the upper body, because these first exercises require more mental and physical energy. The core muscles of the torso are trained before the shoulder and arm muscles that assist them. Exercises often alternate between "pushing" and "pulling" movements to allow their specific supporting muscles time to recover. The stabilizing muscles in the waist should be trained last.

Advanced Techniques

A number of techniques have been developed to make weight training exercises more intense, and thereby potentially increase the rate of progress. Many weight lifters use these techniques to bring themselves past a plateau, a duration where a weightlifter may be unable to do more lifting repetitions, sets, or use higher weight resistance.

Set Structure

Drop Sets

A drop set is an easy method of strength training where you perform a set of any exercise to failure or right before failure, and then reduce the weight and continue to lift for more repetitions with the decreased weight.

Pyramid Sets

Pyramid sets are weight training sets in which the progression is from lighter weights with a greater number of repetitions in the first set, to heavier weights with fewer repetitions in subsequent sets.

A reverse pyramid is the opposite in which the heavier weights are used at the beginning and progressively lightened.

Burnouts

Burnouts combine pyramids and drop sets, working up to higher weights with low reps and then back down to lower weights and high reps.There are a few different ways one could perform burnout sets but the main idea is to perform an exercise until failure. You should start with a weight that is 75% of the amount of the maximum amount of weight you can lift for 1 rep. Once you've performed the exercise to exhaustion, reduce the weight and perform another set until failure, which will usually consist of much fewer repetitions. Burnout sets sound very similar to supersets but there are differences in the results they produce. Supersets help increase muscle mass, but are more efficient for producing muscle definition and shape. Burnout sets help increase muscle growth because of the buildup of lactic acid in the muscle when it's forced to the point of failure.

Diminishing Set

The diminishing set method is where a weight is chosen that can be lifted for 20 reps in one set, and then 70 repetitions are performed in as few sets as possible.

Rest-pause

The rest-pause training method takes one whole set and breaks it down into a few mini sets. There are two different goals that are associated with rest-pause training, you could use it to increase hypertrophy or increase strength. To increase hypertrophy you would perform a set with weight you are comfortable lifting for 6-10 reps and then set the weight down. Next, take 15 seconds worth of deep breaths and pick the weight back up and lift to failure. Lastly, repeat step two as many times as you want but it is commonly done twice. In order to increase strength using rest-pause method first you would choose a weight that is 85-95% of your one rep max. Then you would perform 1 rep with this weight and follow that up with a 30-45 second break. Then you could repeat this process as many times as you'd like.

Giant Set

The Giant set, is a form of training that targets one muscle group (e.g. the triceps) with four separate exercises performed in quick succession, often to failure and sometimes with the reduction of weight halfway through a set once muscle fatigue sets in. This form of intense training 'shocks' the muscles and as such, is usually performed by experienced trainers and should be used infrequently.

Combined Sets

Supersets: Supersets combine two or more exercises with similar motions to maximize the amount of work of an individual muscle or group of muscles. The exercises are performed with no rest period between the exercises. An example would be doing bench press, which predominantly works the pectoralis and triceps muscles, and then moving to an exercise that works just the triceps such as the triceps extension or the pushdown.

Push-pull supersets: Push-pull supersets are similar to regular supersets, but exercises are chosen which work opposing muscle groups. This is especially popular when applied to arm exercises, for example by combining biceps curls with the triceps pushdown. Other examples include the shoulder press and lat pulldown combination, and the bench press and wide grip row combination. A calisthenic example is alternating between pull-ups and dips.

Pre-exhaustion: Pre-exhaustion combines an isolation exercise with a compound exercise for the same muscle group. The isolation exercise first exhausts the muscle group, and then the compound exercise uses the muscle group's supporting muscles to push it further than would otherwise be possible. For example, the triceps muscles normally help the pectorals perform their function. But in the "bench press" the weaker triceps often fails first, which limits the impact on the pectorals. By preceding the bench press with the pec fly, the pectorals can be pre-exhausted so that both muscles fail at the same time, and both benefit equally from the exercise.

Breakdowns: Breakdowns were developed by Frederick Hatfield and Mike Quinn to work the different types of muscle fibers for maximum stimulation. Three different exercises that work the same muscle group are selected, and used for a superset. The first exercise uses a heavy weight (~85% of 1 rep max) for around five reps, the second a medium weight (~70% of 1 rep max) for around twelve reps, and finally the third exercise is performed with a light weight (~50% of 1 rep max) for twenty to thirty reps, or even lighter (~40% of 1 rep max) for forty or more reps. (Going to failure is discouraged.) The entire superset is performed three times.

Beyond Failure

Forced reps: Forced reps occur after momentary muscular failure. An assistant provides just enough help to get the weight trainer past the sticking point of the exercise, and allow further repetitions to be completed. Weight trainers often do this when they are spotting their exercise partner. With some exercises forced reps can be done without a training partner. For example, with one-arm *biceps curls* the other arm can be used to assist the arm that is being trained.

Cheat reps: Cheating is a deliberate compromise of form to maximize reps. Cheating has the advantage that it can be done without a training partner, but compromises safety. A typical example of cheat reps occurs during biceps curls when, beginning with the load at the waist, the exerciser swings the barbell or dumbbell forward and up during the concentric phase utilizing momentum to assist their bicep muscles in moving the load to a shortened muscle position. Momentum assistance during the concentric phase allows them to move greater loads during the more difficult concentric phase. The objective can be to position greater loads of resistance to the biceps in preparation of performing the eccentric phase than the more difficult concentric phase would otherwise allow. Replacing a typical function of a training partner with a solo exerciser performing cheat reps facilitates forced reps or negative reps when training alone.

Weight stripping a.k.a. Number Setting: Weight stripping is a technique used after failure with a normal resistance in certain exercises, particularly with easily adjustable machines, whereby the weight trainer or a partner gradually reduces the resistance after a full set is taken to failure. With each reduction in resistance, as many possible reps are completed and the resistance is then reduced again. This is continued until the resistance is approximately half the original resistance.

Negative reps: Negative reps are performed with much heavier weights. Assistants lift the weight, and then the weight trainer attempts to resist its downward progress through an eccentric contraction. Alternatively, an individual can use an exercise machine for negatives by lifting the weight with both arms or legs, and then lowering it with only one. Or they can simply lower weights more slowly than they lift them: for example, by taking two seconds to lift each weight and four seconds to lower it.

Partial reps: Partial reps, as the name implies, involves movement through only part of the normal path of an exercise. Partial reps can be performed with heavier weights. Usually, only the easiest part of the repetition is attempted.

Burns: Burns involve mixing partial reps into a set of full range reps in order to increase intensity. The partials can be performed at any part of the exercise movement, depending on what works best for the particular exercise. Also, the partials can either be added after the end of a set or in some alternating fashion with the full range reps. For example, after performing a set of *biceps curls* to failure, an individual would cheat the bar back to the most contracted position, and then perform several partial reps.

Other Techniques

Progressive movement training: Progressive movement training attempts to gradually increase the range of motion throughout a training cycle. The lifter will start with a much heavier weight than they could handle in the full range of motion, only moving through the last 3–5" of the movement. Throughout the training cycle, the lifter will gradually increase the range of motion until the joint moves through the full range of the exercise. This is a style that was made popular by Paul Anderson.

Time under tension: Time under tension or TUT repetitions are performed with lighter weights. Time under tension refers to the amount of time your muscle under stress during a set. This consists of the time spent in the concentric or the shortening phase, peak contraction phase, as well as the eccentric or the lengthening phase. For example, if you go perform a set of 10 reps and each rep takes 3 seconds to complete, your muscle is under tension for a total of 30 seconds. If you were to perform the same exercise but if you spent 2 seconds in the concentric phase, 1 second to stop during peak contraction, and 3 seconds to lower the weight during the eccentric phase of the rep, the same 10 reps would end up putting your muscles under tension for about 60 seconds.

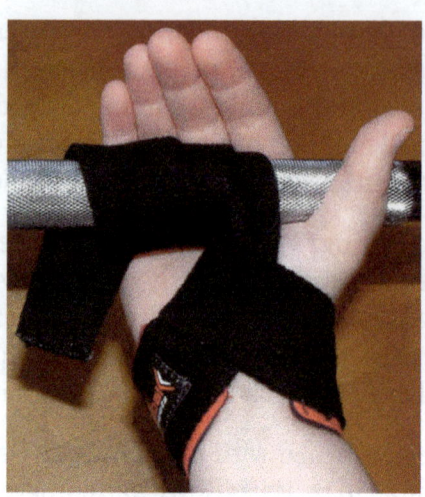

Using a wrist strap.

Wrist straps: Wrist straps (lifting straps) are sometimes used to assist in gripping very heavy weights. Wrist straps can be used to isolate muscle groups like in "lat pull-downs", where the trainee would primarily use the latissimus dorsi muscles of the back rather than the biceps. They are particularly useful for the *deadlift*. Some lifters avoid using wrist straps to develop their grip strength, just as some go further by using thick bars. Wrist straps can allow a lifter initially to use more weight than they might be able to handle safely for an entire set, as unlike simply holding a weight, if it is dropped then the lifter must descend with it or be pulled down. Straps place stress on the bones of the wrist which can be potentially harmful if excessive.

Combined Techniques

Strength training may involve the combining of different training methods such as weight training, plyometrics, bodyweight exercises, and ballistic exercises. This is often done in order to improve a person's ability to apply their strength quickly. Or in other words, to improve their ability to apply explosive power.

Loaded Plyometrics

Loaded plyometrics involve the addition of weights to jumping exercises. The weights may be held or worn. For instance, vertical jumps whilst holding a trap bar or jumping split squats whilst holding dumbbells. This helps to enhance the explosive power of the athlete.

Complex Training

Complex training, also known as contrast training, involves the alternation of weight training and plyometric exercises. Ideally, both sets of exercises should move through similar ranges of movement; such a pairing is called a complex, or contrast, pair. For instance, a set of heavy back squats at about 85-95% 1RM followed by a set of jumping exercises. The intention is to utilise the intense nervous system activation and increased muscle fibre recruitment from the heavy lift in the plyometric exercise; thereby increasing the power with which it can be performed. Over a period of training, this may result in the athlete being able to perform the plyometric exercise more powerfully, without the requirement of the preceding heavy lift. Working on the same principles, a sports specific action may be incorporated instead of the plyometric exercise; the intention, in this case, being to increase the athlete's ability to perform the sports specific action more powerfully.

Ballistic Training

Ballistic training, sometimes referred to as power training, is based upon the principle of maximising the acceleration phase of the exercise and minimising the deceleration phase; this helps to improve the athlete's explosive power. On this basis, ballistic training may include exercises which involve the throwing of a weight, such as a medicine ball, or jumping whilst holding or wearing a weight.

Contrast Loading

Contrast loading is the alternation of heavy and light loads i.e. a heavy bench press set at about 85-95% 1RM followed by a light bench press set at about 30-60% 1RM. The heavy set should be performed fast with the light set being performed as fast as possible. The joints should not be locked as this inhibits muscle fibre recruitment and reduces the speed at which the exercise can be performed. A loaded plyometric exercise, or ballistic exercise, may take the place of the light lift.

Similarly to complex training, contrast loading relies on the intense nervous system activation and enhanced muscle fibre recruitment from the heavy lift to help improve the power with which the subsequent exercise can be performed. This physiological effect is commonly referred to as post-activation potentiation, or the PAP effect. By way of explanation, if a light weight is lifted, and then a heavy weight is lifted, and then the same light weight is lifted again, then the light weight will feel lighter the second time it is lifted. This is due to the increased PAP effect from the heavy lift allowing for greater power to be applied and thus making the subsequent lighter lift feel even lighter than before. Explosive power training programmes are frequently designed to specifically utilise the PAP effect.

Risks and Concerns

Strength training is a safe form of exercise when the movements are controlled, and carefully defined. Some safety measures can also be taken before the training. However, as with any form of exercise, improper execution and the failure to take appropriate precautions can result in injury. A helmet, boots, gloves, and back belt can aide in injury prevention. Principles of weight training safety apply to strength training.

Bodybuilding

Bodybuilding is a sport in which the goal is to increase muscle size and definition. Bodybuilding increases the endurance of muscles, as well as strength, though not as much as if they were the primary goals. Bodybuilders compete in bodybuilding competitions, and use specific principles and methods of strength training to maximize muscular size and develop extremely low levels of body fat. In contrast, most strength trainers train to improve their strength and endurance while not giving special attention to reducing body fat below normal. Strength trainers tend to focus on compound exercises to build basic strength, whereas bodybuilders often use isolation exercises to visually separate their muscles, and to improve muscular symmetry. Pre-contest training for bodybuilders is different again, in that they attempt to retain as much muscular tissue as possible while undergoing severe dieting. However, the bodybuilding community has been the source of many strength training principles, techniques, vocabulary, and customs.

Nutrition

It is widely accepted that strength training must be matched by changes in diet in order to be effective. Although, aerobic exercise has been proven to have an effect on the dietary intake of macronutrients, strength training has not and an increase in dietary protein is generally believed to be required for building skeletal muscle.

Research studies found that supplementation of protein in the diet of healthy adults increased the size and strength of muscles during prolonged resistance exercise training; protein intakes of greater than 1.6 g/kg/day did not additionally increase fat-free mass or muscle size or strength. Protein that is neither needed for cell growth and repair nor consumed for energy is converted into urea mainly through the deamination process and is excreted by the kidneys. It was once thought that a high-protein diet entails risk of kidney damage, but studies have shown that kidney problems only occur in people with previous kidney disease. However, failure to properly hydrate can put an increased strain on the kidney's ability to function. An adequate supply of carbohydrates (5–7 g per kg) is also needed as a source of energy and for the body to restore glycogen levels in muscles.

A light, balanced meal prior to the workout (usually one to two hours beforehand) ensures that adequate energy and amino acids are available for the intense bout of exercise. The type of nutrients consumed affects the response of the body, and nutrient timing whereby protein and carbohydrates are consumed prior to and after workout has a beneficial impact on muscle growth. Water is consumed throughout the course of the workout to prevent poor performance due to dehydration. A protein shake is often consumed immediately following the workout, because both protein uptake and protein usage are increased at this time. Glucose (or another simple sugar) is often consumed as well since this quickly replenishes any glycogen lost during the exercise period. To maximise muscle protein anabolism, recovery drink should contain glucose (dextrose), protein (usually whey) hydrolysate containing mainly dipeptides and tripeptides, and leucine. Some weight trainers also take ergogenic aids such as creatine or steroids to aid muscle growth. However, the effectiveness of some products is disputed and others are potentially harmful.

Sex Differences in Mass Gains

Due to the androgenic hormonal differences between males and females, the latter are generally unable to develop large muscles regardless of the training program used. Normally the most that can be achieved is a look similar to that of a fitness model. Muscle is denser than fat, so someone who builds muscle while keeping the same body weight will occupy less volume; if two people weigh the same (and are the same height) but have different lean body mass percentages, the one with more muscle will appear thinner.

In addition, though bodybuilding uses the same principles as strength training, it is with a goal of gaining muscle bulk. Strength trainers with different goals and programs will not gain the same mass as a professional bodybuilder.

Muscle Toning

Some weight trainers perform light, high-repetition exercises in an attempt to "tone" their muscles without increasing their size. In anatomy and physiology, as well as medicine, the term "muscle tone" refers to the continuous and passive partial contraction of the muscles, or the muscles' resistance to passive stretching during resting state as determined by a deep tendon reflex. Muscle tonus is dependent on neurological input into the muscle. In medicine, observations of changes in muscle tonus can be used to determine normal or abnormal states which can be indicative of pathology. The common strength training term "tone" is derived from this use.

What muscle builders refer to as a *toned physique* or "muscle firmness" is one that combines reasonable muscular size with moderate levels of body fat, qualities that may result from a combination of diet and exercise.

Muscle tone or firmness is derived from the increase in actin and myosin cross filaments in the sarcomere. When this occurs the same amount of neurological input creates a greater firmness or tone in the resting continuous and passive partial contraction in the muscle.

Exercises of 6–12 reps cause hypertrophy of the sarcoplasm in slow-twitch and high-twitch muscle fibers, contributing to overall increased muscle bulk. This is not to be confused with myofibril hypertrophy which leads to strength gains. Both however can occur to an extent during this rep range. Even though most are of the opinion that higher repetitions are best for producing the desired effect of muscle firmness or tone, it is not. Low volume strength training of 5 repetitions or fewer will increase strength by increasing actin and myosin cross filaments thereby increasing muscle firmness or tone. The low volume of this training will inhibit the hypertrophy effect.

Lowered-calorie diets have no positive effect on muscle hypertrophy for muscle of any fiber type. They may, however, decrease the thickness of subcutaneous fat (fat between muscle and skin), through an overall reduction in body fat, thus making muscle striations more visible.

Weight Loss

Exercises like sit-ups, or abdominal crunches, performs less work than whole-body aerobic exercises thereby expending fewer calories during exercise than jogging, for example.

Hypertrophy serves to maintain muscle mass, for an elevated basal metabolic rate, which has the potential to burn more calories in a given period compared to aerobics. This helps to maintain a higher metabolic rate which would otherwise diminish after metabolic adaption to dieting, or upon completion of an aerobic routine.

Weight loss also depends on the type of strength training used. Weight training is generally used for bulking, but the bulking method will more than likely not increase weight because of the diet involved. However, when resistance or circuit training is used, because they are not geared towards bulking, women tend to lose weight more quickly. Lean muscles require calories to maintain themselves at rest, which will help reduce fat through an increase in the basal metabolic rate.

Bodyweight Exercise

Bodyweight exercises are strength training exercises that use the individual's own weight to provide resistance against gravity. Bodyweight exercises can enhance a range of biomotor abilities including strength, power, endurance, speed, flexibility, coordination and balance. This type of strength training has grown in popularity for both recreational and professional athletes. Bodyweight training utilises simple abilities such as pushing, pulling, squatting, bending, twisting and balancing. Movements such as the push-up, the pull-up, and the sit-up are some of the most common bodyweight exercises.

Advantages

While some exercises may require some type of equipment, the majority of bodyweight exercises require none. For those exercises that do require equipment, common items found in the household are usually sufficient (such as a bath towel for towel curls), or substitutes can usually be improvised (for example, using a horizontal tree branch to perform pull ups). Therefore, bodyweight exercises are convenient when travelling or on vacation, when access to a gym or specialised equipment may not be possible. Another advantage of bodyweight training is that there are no costs involved.

Disadvantages

As bodyweight exercises use the individual's own weight to provide the resistance for the movement, the weight being lifted is never greater than the weight of one's own body. Another disadvantage is that bodyweight training may be daunting to novices and seen to be too easy for experienced athletes. Women, in general, also find it more difficult to do bodyweight exercises involving upper body strength and may be discouraged from undertaking these exercises in their fitness regimens.

Bodyweight Exercise for Older Adults

Some bodyweight exercises have been shown to benefit not just the young, but the elderly as well. Older people undertaking bodyweight exercises benefit through increased muscle mass, increased mobility, increased bone density, decreased depression and improved sleep habits. It is also believed that bodyweight training may assist in decreasing or even preventing cognitive decline as people age. In addition, the increased risk of falls seen in elderly people can be mitigated by bodyweight training. Exercises focusing on the legs and abdomen such as squats, lunges and step ups are recommended to increase leg and core strength and, in doing so, reduce fall risk. These bodyweight exercises provide multi-directional movement that mimics daily activities, and can thus be preferable to using weight machines.

Weight Training

Weight training is a common type of strength training for developing the strength and size of skeletal muscles. It utilizes the force of gravity in the form of weighted bars, dumbbells or weight stacks in order to oppose the force generated by muscle through concentric or eccentric contraction. Weight training uses a variety of specialized equipment to target specific muscle groups and types of movement.

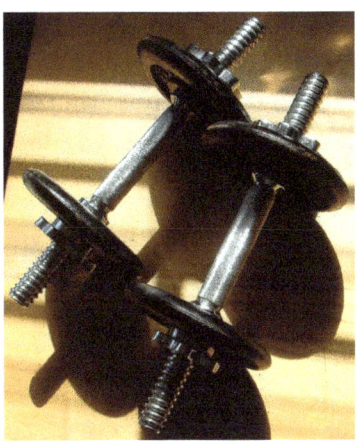

A complete weight training workout can be performed with a pair of
adjustable dumbbells and a set of weight disks (plates).

Sports for which strength training is central are bodybuilding, weightlifting, powerlifting, strong-man, highland games, hammer throw, shot put, discus throw, and javelin throw. Many other sports use strength training as part of their training regimen, notably: American football, baseball, basketball, cricket, football, hockey, lacrosse, mixed martial arts, rowing, rugby league, rugby union, track and field, boxing and wrestling.

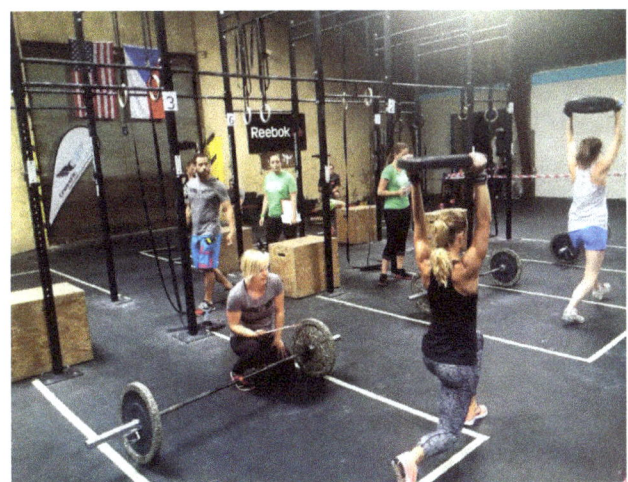

Weight training can be incorporated into numerous fitness regimes.

The basic principles of weight training are essentially identical to those of strength training, and involve a manipulation of the number of repetitions (reps), sets, tempo, exercise types, and weight moved to cause desired increases in strength, endurance, and size. The specific combinations of reps, sets, exercises, and weights depends on the aims of the individual performing the exercise.

In addition to the basic principles of *strength training*, a further consideration added by weight training is the equipment used. Types of equipment include barbells, dumbbells, kettlebells, pulleys and stacks in the form of weight machines, and the body's own weight in the case of chin-ups and push-ups. Different types of weights will give different types of resistance, and often the same absolute weight can have different relative weights depending on the type of equipment used. For example, lifting 10 kilograms using a dumbbell sometimes requires more force than moving 10 kilograms on a weight stack if certain pulley arrangements are used. In other cases, the weight stack may require more force than the equivalent dumbbell weight due to additional torque or resistance in the machine. Additionally, although they may display the same weight stack, different machines may be heavier or lighter depending on the number of pulleys and their arrangements.

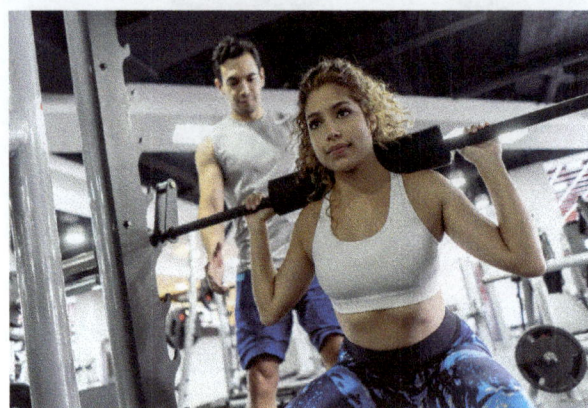

A woman doing weight training at a health club with her coach standing behind her.

Weight training also requires the use of proper or 'good form', performing the movements with the appropriate muscle group, and not transferring the weight to different body parts in order to move greater weight (called 'cheating'). Failure to use good form during a training set can result in injury or a failure to meet training goals. If the desired muscle group is not challenged sufficiently, the threshold of overload is never reached and the muscle does not gain in strength. At a particularly advanced level; however, "cheating" can be used to break through strength plateaus and encourage neurological and muscular adaptation.

Safety

Weight training is a safe form of exercise when the movements are controlled and carefully defined. However, as with any form of exercise, improper execution and the failure to take appropriate precautions can result in injury.

Maintaining Proper Form

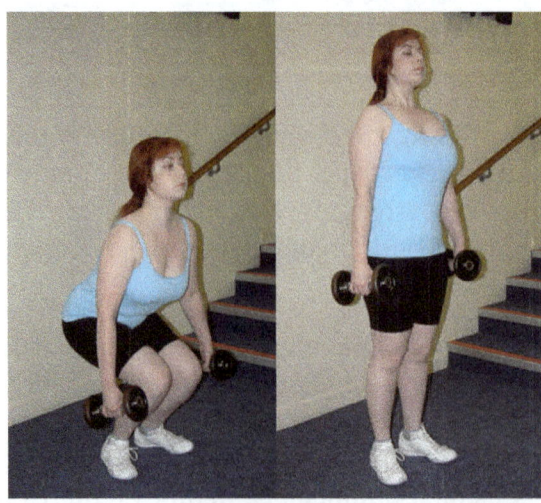

A dumbbell half-squat.

Maintaining proper form is one of the many steps in order to perfectly perform a certain technique. Correct form in weight training improves strength, muscle tone, and maintaining a healthy weight. Proper form will prevent any strains or fractures. When the exercise becomes difficult towards the end of a set, there is a temptation to cheat, i.e., to use poor form to recruit other muscle groups to assist the effort. Avoid heavy weight and keep the number of repetitions to a minimum. This may shift the effort to weaker muscles that cannot handle the weight. For example, the *squat* and the *deadlift* are used to exercise the largest muscles in the body—the leg and buttock muscles—so they require substantial weight. Beginners are tempted to round their back while performing these exercises. The relaxation of the spinal erectors which allows the lower back to round can cause shearing in the vertebrae of the lumbar spine, potentially damaging the spinal discs.

Stretching and Warm-up

Weight trainers commonly spend 5 to 20 minutes warming up their muscles before starting a workout. It is common to stretch the entire body to increase overall flexibility; many people stretch just the area being worked that day. It has been observed that static stretching can increase the risk of injury due to its analgesic effect and cellular damage caused by it. A proper warm-up routine, however, has shown to be effective in minimising the chances of injury, especially if they are done with the same movements performed in the weigh lifting exercise. When properly warmed up the lifter will have more strength and stamina since the blood has begun to flow to the muscle groups.

Breathing

In weight training, as with most forms of exercise, there is a tendency for the breathing pattern to deepen. This helps to meet increased oxygen requirements. Holding the breath or breathing shallowly is avoided because it may lead to a lack of oxygen, passing out, or an increase in blood pressure. Generally, the recommended breathing technique is to inhale when lowering the weight (the eccentric portion) and exhale when lifting the weight (the concentric portion). However, the reverse, inhaling when lifting and exhaling when lowering, may also be recommended. Some researchers state that there is little difference between the two techniques in terms of their influence on heart rate and blood pressure. It may also be recommended that a weight lifter simply breathes in a manner which feels appropriate.

Deep breathing may be specifically recommended for the lifting of heavy weights because it helps to generate intra-abdominal pressure which can help to strengthen the posture of the lifter, and especially their core.

In particular situations, a coach may advise performing the valsalva maneuver during exercises which place a load on the spine. The vasalva maneuver consists of closing the windpipe and clenching the abdominal muscles as if exhaling, and is performed naturally and unconsciously by most people when applying great force. It serves to stiffen the abdomen and torso and assist the back muscles and spine in supporting the heavy weight. Although it briefly increases blood pressure, its is still recommended by weightlifting experts such as Rippetoe since the risk of a stroke by aneurysm is far lower than the risk of an orthopedic injury caused by inadequate rigidity of the torso. Some medical experts warn that the mechanism of building "high levels of intra-abdominal pressure (IAP) produced by breath holding using the Valsava maneuver", to "ensure spine stiffness and stability during these extraordinary demands", "should be considered only for extreme weight-lifting challenges — not for rehabilitation exercise".

Hydration

As with other sports, weight trainers should avoid dehydration throughout the workout by drinking sufficient water. This is particularly true in hot environments, or for those older than 65.

Some athletic trainers advise athletes to drink about 7 imperial fluid ounces (200 mL) every 15 minutes while exercising, and about 80 imperial fluid ounces (2.3 L) throughout the day.

However, a much more accurate determination of how much fluid is necessary can be made by performing appropriate weight measurements before and after a typical exercise session, to determine how much fluid is lost during the workout. The greatest source of fluid loss during exercise is through perspiration, but as long as your fluid intake is roughly equivalent to your rate of perspiration, hydration levels will be maintained.

Under most circumstances, sports drinks do not offer a physiological benefit over water during weight training. However, high-intensity exercise for a continuous duration of at least one hour may require the replenishment of electrolytes which a sports drink may provide. 'Sports drinks' that contain simple carbohydrates & water do not cause ill effects, but are most likely unnecessary for the average trainee.

Insufficient hydration may cause lethargy, soreness or muscle cramps. The urine of well-hydrated persons should be nearly colorless, while an intense yellow color is normally a sign of insufficient hydration.

Avoiding Pain

An exercise should be halted if marked or sudden pain is felt, to prevent further injury. However, not all discomfort indicates injury. Weight training exercises are brief but very intense, and many people are unaccustomed to this level of effort. The expression "no pain, no gain" refers to working through the discomfort expected from such vigorous effort, rather than to willfully ignore extreme pain, which may indicate serious soft tissue injuries. The focus must be proper form, not the amount of weight lifted.

Discomfort can arise from other factors. Individuals who perform large numbers of repetitions, sets, and exercises for each muscle group may experience a burning sensation in their muscles. These individuals may also experience a swelling sensation in their muscles from increased blood flow also known as edema (the "pump"). True muscle fatigue is experienced as loss of power in muscles due to a lack of ATP, the energy used by our body, or a marked and uncontrollable loss of strength in a muscle, arising from the nervous system (motor unit) rather than from the muscle fibers themselves. Extreme neural fatigue can be experienced as temporary muscle failure. Some weight training programs, such as Metabolic Resistance Training, actively seek temporary muscle failure; evidence to support this type of training is mixed at best. Irrespective of their program, however, most athletes engaged in high-intensity weight training will experience muscle failure during their regimens.

Beginners are advised to build up slowly to a weight training program. Untrained individuals may have some muscles that are comparatively stronger than others; nevertheless, an injury can result if (in a particular exercise) the primary muscle is stronger than its stabilizing muscles. Building up slowly allows muscles time to develop appropriate strengths relative to each other. This can also help to minimize delayed onset muscle soreness. A sudden start to an intense program can cause significant muscular soreness. Unexercised muscles contain cross-linkages that are torn during intense exercise. A regimen of flexibility exercises should be implemented before and after workouts. Since weight training puts great strain on the muscles, it is necessary to warm-up properly. Kinetic stretching before a workout and static stretching after are a key part of flexibility and injury prevention.

Other Precautions

Anyone beginning an intensive physical training program is typically advised to consult a physician, because of possible undetected heart or other conditions for which such activity is contraindicated.

Exercises like the bench press or the squat in which a failed lift can potentially result in the lifter becoming trapped under the weight are normally performed inside a power rack or in the presence of one or more spotters, who can safely re-rack the barbell if the weight trainer is unable to do so. In addition to spotters, knowledge of proper form and the use of safety bars can go a long way to keep a lifter from suffering injury due to a failed repetition.

Equipment

Weight training usually requires different types of equipment, most commonly dumbbells, barbells, weight plates, and weight machines. Various combinations of specific exercises, machines, dumbbells, and barbells allow trainees to exercise body parts in numerous ways.

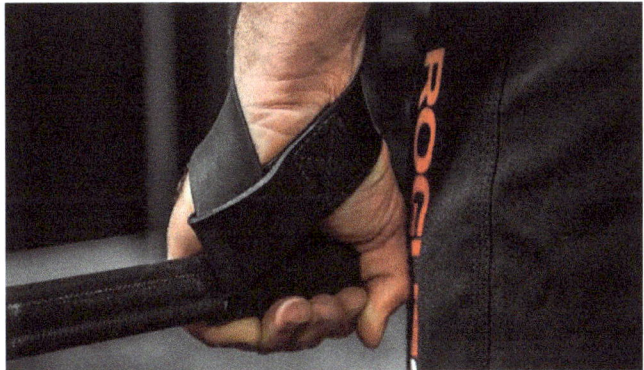

A lifting strap.

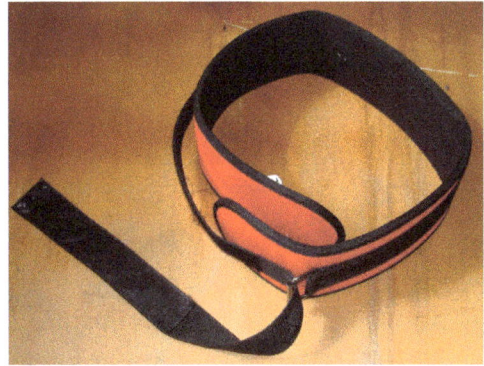

A lifting belt.

Other types of equipment include:

- Lifting straps, which allow more weight to be lifted by transferring the load to the wrists and avoiding limitations in forearm muscles and grip strength.

- Weightlifting belts, which are meant to brace the core through intra-abdominal pressure.

Controversy exists regarding the safety of these devices and their proper use is often mis-understood.

- Weighted clothing, bags of sand, lead shot, or other materials that are strapped to wrists, ankles, torso or other body parts to increase the amount of work required by muscles.

- Gloves can improve grip, prevent the formation of calluses on the hands, relieve pressure on the wrists, and provide support.

- Chalk ($MgCO_3$), which dries out sweaty hands, improving grip.

- Wrist and knee wraps.

- Shoes, which have a flat, rigid sole to provide a sturdy base of support, and may feature a raised heel of varying height (usually 0.5" or 0.75") to accommodate a lifter's biomechanics for more efficient squats, deadlifts, overhead presses, and Olympic lifts.

Types of Exercises

Isolation Exercises versus Compound Exercises

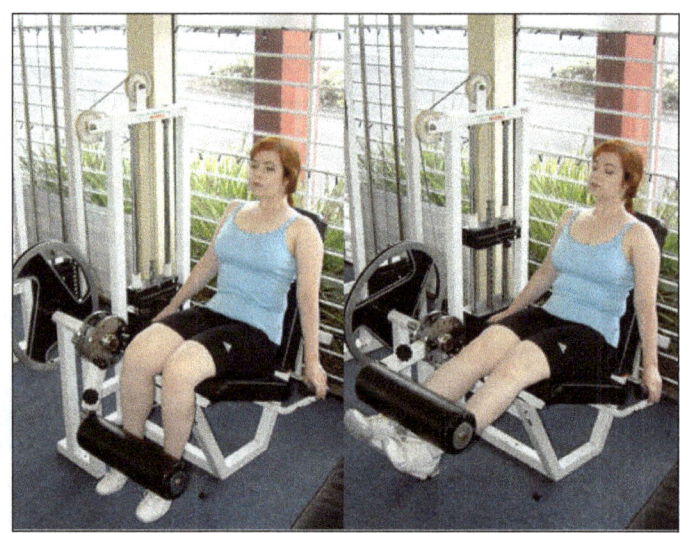
The leg extension is an isolation exercise.

An isolation exercise is one where the movement is restricted to one joint only. For example, the *leg extension* is an isolation exercise for the quadriceps. Specialized types of equipment are used to ensure that other muscle groups are only minimally involved—they just help the individual maintain a stable posture—and movement occurs only around the knee joint. Isolation exercises involve machines, dumbbells, barbells (free weights), and pulley machines. Pulley machines and free weights can be used when combined with special/proper positions and joint bracing.

Compound exercises work several muscle groups at once, and include movement around two or more joints. For example, in the *leg press*, movement occurs around the hip, knee and ankle joints. This exercise is primarily used to develop the quadriceps, but it also involves the hamstrings, glutes and calves. Compound exercises are generally similar to the ways that people naturally push, pull and lift objects, whereas isolation exercises often feel a little unnatural.

Each type of exercise has its uses. Compound exercises build the basic strength that is needed to perform everyday pushing, pulling and lifting activities. Isolation exercises are useful for "rounding out" a routine, by directly exercising muscle groups that cannot be fully exercised in the compound exercises.

The type of exercise performed also depends on the individual's goals. Those who seek to increase their performance in sports would focus mostly on compound exercises, with isolation exercises being used to strengthen just those muscles that are holding the athlete back. Similarly, a power-lifter would focus on the specific compound exercises that are performed at powerlifting competitions. However, those who seek to improve the look of their body without necessarily maximizing their strength gains (including bodybuilders) would put more of an emphasis on isolation exercises. Both types of athletes, however, generally make use of both compound and isolation exercises.

Free Weights versus Weight Machines

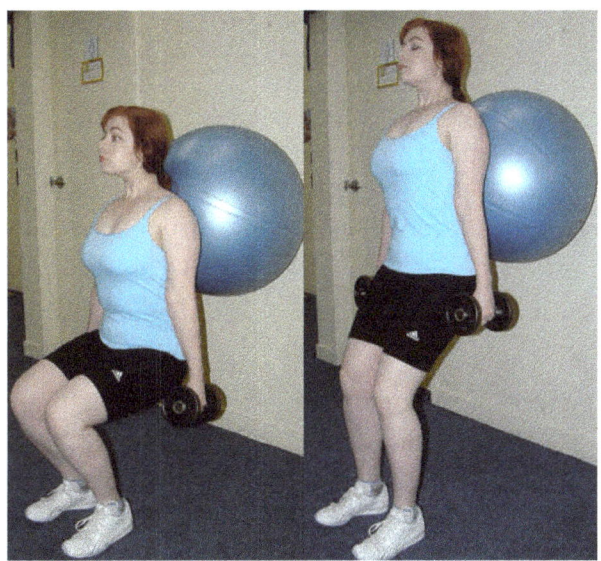

Exercise balls allow a wider range of free weight exercises to be performed. They are also known as Swiss balls, stability balls, fitness balls, gym balls, sports balls, therapy balls or body balls. They are sometimes confused with medicine balls.

Free weights include dumbbells, barbells, medicine balls, sandbells, and kettlebells. Unlike weight machines, they do not constrain users to specific, fixed movements, and therefore require more effort from the individual's stabilizer muscles. It is often argued that free weight exercises are superior for precisely this reason. For example, they are recommended for golf players, since golf is a unilateral exercise that can break body balances, requiring exercises to keep the balance in muscles.

Some free weight exercises can be performed while sitting or lying on an exercise ball.

There are a number of weight machines that are commonly found in neighborhood gyms. The Smith machine is a barbell that is constrained to vertical movement. The cable machine consists of two weight stacks separated by 2.5 metres, with cables running through adjustable pulleys (that can be fixed at any height so as to select different amounts of weight) to various types of handles. There are also exercise-specific weight machines such as the leg press. A multigym includes a variety of exercise-specific mechanisms in one apparatus.

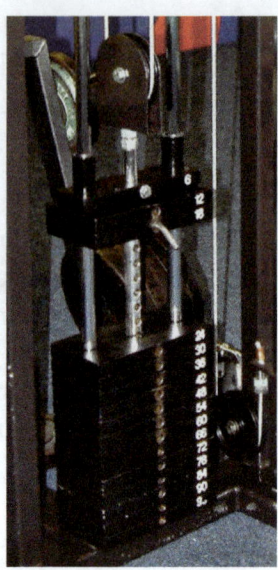

The weight stack from a cable machine.

One limitation of many free weight exercises and exercise machines is that the muscle is working maximally against gravity during only a small portion of the lift. Some exercise-specific machines feature an oval cam (first introduced by Nautilus) which varies the resistance, so that the resistance, and the muscle force required, remains constant throughout the full range of motion of the exercise.

Push-pull Workout

A push–pull workout is a method of arranging a weight training routine so that exercises alternate between push motions and pull motions. A push–pull superset is two complementary segments (one pull/one push) done back-to-back. An example is bench press (push) / bent-over row (pull). Another push–pull technique is to arrange workout routines so that one day involves only push (usually chest, shoulders and triceps) exercises, and an alternate day only pull (usually back and biceps) exercises so the body can get adequate rest.

Isotonic and Plyometric Exercises

These terms combine the prefix *iso-* (meaning "same") with *tonic* ("strength") and *plio-* ("more") with *metric* ("distance"). In "isotonic" exercises the force applied to the muscle does not change (while the length of the muscle decreases or increases) while in "plyometric" exercises the length of the muscle stretches and contracts rapidly to increase the power output of a muscle.

Weight training is primarily an isotonic form of exercise, as the force produced by the muscle to push or pull weighted objects should not change (though in practice the force produced does decrease as muscles fatigue). Any object can be used for weight training, but dumbbells, barbells, and other specialised equipment are normally used because they can be adjusted to specific weights and are easily gripped. Many exercises are not strictly isotonic because the force on the muscle varies as the joint moves through its range of motion. Movements can become easier or harder depending on the angle of muscular force relative to gravity; for example, a standard biceps curl becomes easier as the hand approaches the shoulder as more of the load is taken by the structure of the elbow. Originating from Nautilus, Inc., some machines use a logarithmic-spiral cam to keep resistance constant irrespective of the joint angle.

Plyometrics exploit the stretch-shortening cycle of muscles to enhance the myotatic (stretch) reflex. This involves rapid alternation of lengthening and shortening of muscle fibers against resistance. The resistance involved is often a weighted object such as a medicine ball or sandbag, but can also be the body itself as in jumping exercises or the body with a weight vest that allows movement with resistance. Plyometrics is used to develop explosive speed, and focuses on maximal power instead of maximal strength by compressing the force of muscular contraction into as short a period as possible, and may be used to improve the effectiveness of a boxer's punch, or to increase the vertical jumping ability of a basketball player. Care must be taken when performing plyometric exercises because they inflict greater stress upon the involved joints and tendons than other forms of exercise.

Health Benefits

Benefits of weight training include increased strength, muscle mass, endurance, bone and bone mineral density, insulin sensitivity, GLUT 4 density, HDL cholesterol, improved cardiovascular health and appearance, and decreased body fat, blood pressure, LDL cholesterol and triglycerides.

The body's basal metabolic rate increases with increases in muscle mass, which promotes long-term fat loss and helps dieters avoid yo-yo dieting. Moreover, intense workouts elevate metabolism for several hours following the workout, which also promotes fat loss.

Weight training also provides functional benefits. Stronger muscles improve posture, provide better support for joints, and reduce the risk of injury from everyday activities. Older people who take up weight training can prevent some of the loss of muscle tissue that normally accompanies aging—and even regain some functional strength—and by doing so, become less frail. They may be able to avoid some types of physical disability. Weight-bearing exercise also helps to prevent osteoporosis. The benefits of weight training for older people have been confirmed by studies of people who began engaging in it even in their eighties and nineties.

For many people in rehabilitation or with an acquired disability, such as following stroke or orthopaedic surgery, strength training for weak muscles is a key factor to optimise recovery. For people with such a health condition, their strength training is likely to need to be designed by an appropriate health professional, such as a physiotherapist.

Stronger muscles improve performance in a variety of sports. Sport-specific training routines are used by many competitors. These often specify that the speed of muscle contraction during weight training should be the same as that of the particular sport. Sport-specific training routines also often include variations to both free weight and machine movements that may not be common for traditional weightlifting.

Though weight training can stimulate the cardiovascular system, many exercise physiologists, based on their observation of maximal oxygen uptake, argue that aerobics training is a better cardiovascular stimulus. Central catheter monitoring during resistance training reveals increased cardiac output, suggesting that strength training shows potential for cardiovascular exercise. However, a 2007 meta-analysis found that, though aerobic training is an effective therapy for heart failure patients, combined aerobic and strength training is ineffective; "the favorable antiremodeling role of aerobic exercise was not confirmed when this mode of exercise was combined with strength training".

One side-effect of any intense exercise is increased levels of dopamine, serotonin and norepinephrine, which can help to improve mood and counter feelings of depression.

Weight training has also been shown to benefit dieters as it inhibits lean body mass loss (as opposed to fat loss) when under a caloric deficit. Weight training also strengthens bones, helping to prevent bone loss and osteoporosis. By increasing muscular strength and improving balance, weight training can also reduce falls by elderly persons. Weight training is also attracting attention for the benefits it can have on the brain, and in older adults, a 2017 meta analysis found that it was effective in improving cognitive performance.

Weight Training and other Types of Strength Training

The benefits of weight training overall are comparable to most other types of strength training: increased muscle, tendon and ligament strength, bone density, flexibility, tone, metabolic rate, and postural support. This type of training will also help prevent injury for athletes. There are benefits and limitations to weight training as compared to other types of strength training. Contrary to popular belief, weight training can be beneficial for both men and women.

Weight Training and Bodybuilding

Although weight training is similar to bodybuilding, they have different objectives. Bodybuilders use weight training to develop their muscles for size, shape, and symmetry regardless of any increase in strength for competition in bodybuilding contests; they train to maximize their muscular size and develop extremely low levels of body fat. In contrast, many weight trainers train to improve their strength and anaerobic endurance while not giving special attention to reducing body fat far below normal.

The bodybuilding community has been the source of many weight training principles, techniques, vocabulary, and customs. Weight training does allow tremendous flexibility in exercises and weights which can allow bodybuilders to target specific muscles and muscle groups, as well as attain specific goals. Not all bodybuilding is undertaken to compete in bodybuilding contests and, in fact, the vast majority of bodybuilders never compete, but bodybuild for their own personal reasons.

Complex Training

In complex training, weight training is typically combined with plyometric exercises in an alternating sequence. Ideally, the weight lifting exercise and the plyometric exercise should move through similar ranges of movement i.e. a back squat at 85-95% 1RM followed by a vertical jump. An advantage of this form of training is that it allows the intense activation of the nervous system and increased muscle fibre recruitment from the weight lifting exercise to be utilized in the subsequent plyometric exercise; thereby improving the power with which it can be performed. Over a period of training, this may enhance the athlete's ability to apply power. The plyometric exercise may be replaced with a sports specific action. The intention being to utilize the neural and muscular activation from the heavy lift in the sports specific action, in order to be able to perform it more powerfully. Over a period of training this may enhance the athlete's ability to perform that sports specific action more powerfully, without a precursory heavy lift being required.

Ballistic Training

Ballistic training incorporates weight training in such a way that the acceleration phase of the movement is maximized and the deceleration phase minimized; thereby increasing the power of the movement overall. For example, throwing a weight or jumping whilst holding a weight. This can be contrasted with a standard weight lifting exercise where there is a distinct deceleration phase at the end of the repetition which stops the weight from moving.

Contrast Loading

Contrast loading is the alternation of heavy and light loads. Considered as sets, the heavy load is performed at about 85-95% 1 repetition max; the light load should be considerably lighter at about 30-60% 1RM. Both sets should be performed fast with the lighter set being performed as fast as possible. The joints should not be locked as this inhibits muscle fibre recruitment and reduces the speed at which the exercise can be performed. The lighter set may be a loaded plyometric exercise such as loaded squat jumps or jumps with a trap bar.

Similarly to complex training, contrast loading relies upon the enhanced activation of the nervous system and increased muscle fibre recruitment from the heavy set, to allow the lighter set to be performed more powerfully. Such a physiological effect is commonly referred to as post-activation potentiation, or the PAP effect. Contrast loading can effectively demonstrate the PAP effect: if a light weight is lifted, and then a heavy weight is lifted, and then the same light weight is lifted again, then the light weight will feel lighter the second time it has been lifted. This is due to the enhanced PAP effect which occurs as a result of the heavy lift being utilised in the subsequent lighter lift; thus making the weight feel lighter and allowing the lift to be performed more powerfully.

Weight Training versus Isometric Training

Isometric exercise provides a maximum amount of resistance based on the force output of the muscle, or muscles pitted against one another. This maximum force maximally strengthens the muscles over all of the joint angles at which the isometric exercise occurs. By comparison, weight training also strengthens the muscle throughout the range of motion the joint is trained in, but only maximally at one angle, causing a lesser increase in physical strength at other angles from the initial through terminating joint angle as compared with isometric exercise. In addition, the risk of injury from weights used in weight training is greater than with isometric exercise (no weights), and the risk of asymmetric training is also greater than with isometric exercise of identical opposing muscles.

Stretching

Stretching is a form of physical exercise in which a specific muscle or tendon (or muscle group) is deliberately flexed or stretched in order to improve the muscle's felt elasticity and achieve comfortable muscle tone. The result is a feeling of increased muscle control, flexibility, and range of motion. Stretching is also used therapeutically to alleviate cramps.

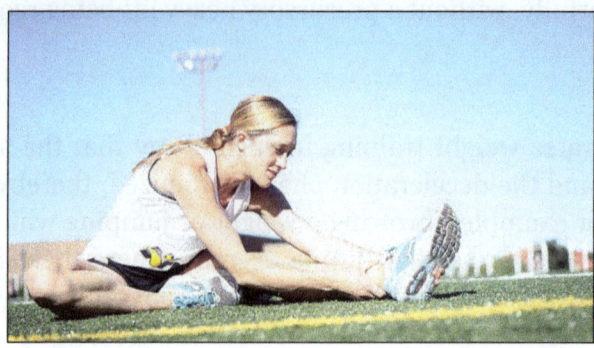

In its most basic form, stretching is a natural and instinctive activity; it is performed by humans and many other animals. It can be accompanied by yawning. Stretching often occurs instinctively after waking from sleep, after long periods of inactivity, or after exiting confined spaces and areas.

Increasing flexibility through stretching is one of the basic tenets of physical fitness. It is common for athletes to stretch before (for warming up) and after exercise in an attempt to reduce risk of injury and increase performance.

Stretching can be dangerous when performed incorrectly. There are many techniques for stretching in general, but depending on which muscle group is being stretched, some techniques may be ineffective or detrimental, even to the point of causing hypermobility, instability, or permanent damage to the tendons, ligaments, and muscle fiber. The physiological nature of stretching and theories about the effect of various techniques are therefore subject to heavy inquiry.

Although static stretching is part of some warm-up routines, a study in 2013 indicated that it weakens muscles. For this reason, an active dynamic warm-up is recommended before exercise in place of static stretching.

Physiology

Studies have shed light on the function, in stretching, of a large protein within the myofibrils of skeletal muscles named titin. A study performed by Magid and Law demonstrated that the origin of passive muscle tension (which occurs during stretching) is actually within the myofibrils, not extracellularly as had previously been supposed. Due to neurological safeguards against injury such as the Golgi tendon reflex, it is normally impossible for adults to stretch most muscle groups to their fullest length without training due to the activation of muscle antagonists as the muscle reaches the limit of its normal range of motion.

Types of Stretches

Stretches can be either static or dynamic, where static stretches are performed while stationary and dynamic stretches involve movement of the muscle during the stretch. Stretches can also be active or passive, where active stretches use internal forces generated by the body to perform a stretch and passive stretches involve forces from external objects or people to facilitate the stretch. Stretches can involve both passive and active components.

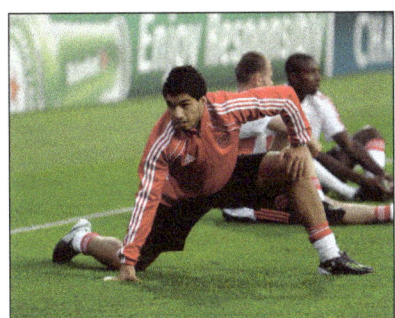

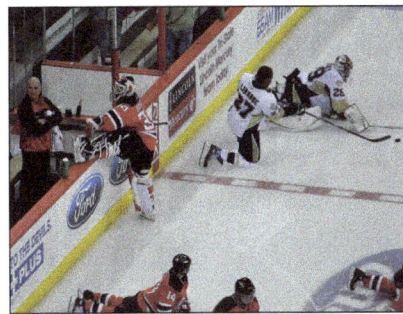

Football player Luis Suárez stretching prior to a match.

Martin Brodeur stretching on the Devils' bench during warmups.

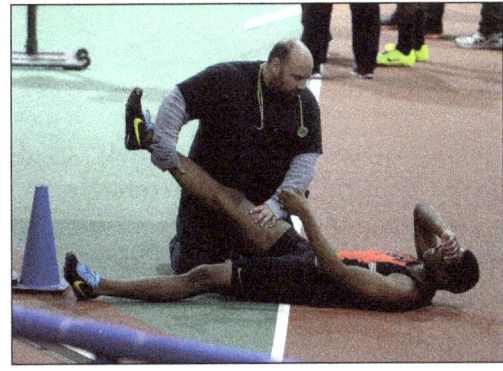

Assisted stretching may be performed when the athlete is unable to stretch optimally independently. For example, during cramping of the hamstrings, assistance in stretching out the muscles may help.

Dynamic Stretching

Dynamic stretching is a movement based stretch aimed on increasing blood flow throughout the body while also loosing up the muscle fibers. Standard dynamic stretches typically involve slow and controlled active contraction of muscles. An example of such a dynamic stretch are lunges. Another form of dynamic stretching is ballistic stretching, which is an active stretch that involves bouncing or swinging back and forth at a high speed in order to take a muscle beyond its typical range of motion using momentum. Ballistic stretching may cause damage to the joints.

Static Stretching

The simplest static stretches are static-passive stretches, which bring the joint to its end range of motion and hold it there using external forces. There are more advanced forms of static stretching, such as proprioceptive neuromuscular facilitation (PNF), which involves both active muscle contractions and passive external forces. PNF stretching may involve contracting either the antagonist muscles, agonist muscles, or both (CRAC).

Effectiveness

Stretching has been found both effective, and ineffective based on its application for treatment.

Although many people engage in stretching before or after exercise, the medical evidence has shown this has no meaningful benefit in preventing specifically muscle soreness.

Stretching does not appear to reduce the risk of injury during exercises, except perhaps for runners. There is some evidence that pre-exercise stretching may increase athletes' range of movement.

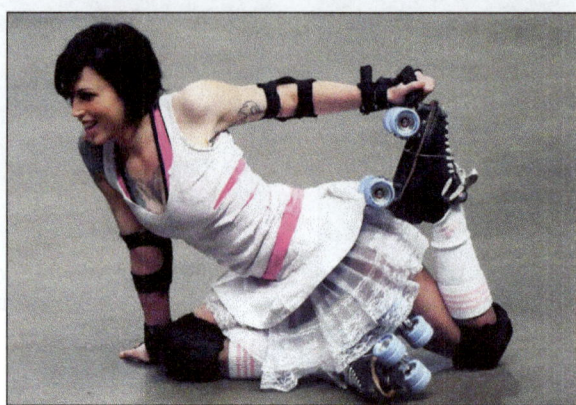

A roller derby athlete stretching.

There are different positives and negatives for the two main types of stretching: static and dynamic. Static stretching is better at creating a more intense stretch because it is able to isolate a muscle group better. But this intense of a stretch may hinder one's athletic performance because the muscle is being over stretched while held in this position and, once the tension is released, the muscle will tend to tighten up and may actually become weaker than it was previously. Also, the longer the duration of static stretching, the more exhausted the muscle becomes. This type of stretching has been shown to have negative results on athletic performance within the categories of power and speed.

Dynamic stretching, because it is movement-based, may not isolate the muscle group as well or have as intense of a stretch, but it is better at increasing the circulation of blood flow throughout the body, which in turn increases the amount of oxygen able to be used for an athletic performance. This type of stretching has shown better results on athletic performances of power and speed, when compared to static stretching.

However, both of these types of stretching have been shown to have a positive impact on flexibility over time by increasing muscle and joint elasticity, thus increasing the depth and range of motion an athlete is able to reach. This is evident in the experiment "Acute effects of duration on sprint performance of adolescent football players." In this experiment, football players were put through different stretching durations of static and dynamic stretching to test their effects. They were tested on maximum sprinting ability and overall change in flexibility. Both static and dynamic stretching had a positive impact on flexibility but, whereas dynamic stretching had no impact on sprint times, static stretching had a negative result, worsening the time the participants were able to sprint the distance in. While the duration of stretching for dynamic had no impact on the overall results, the longer the stretch was held for static, the worse the results got, showing that the longer the duration of stretching held, the weaker the muscle became.

Stretching Tools

- Foam Roller

- BOSU

- Stretch Band

- Flexcushion

Wingate Test

The ergonometer test (also known as the *ergonometer Anaerobic Test (WAnT)*) is an anaerobic exercise test, most often performed on a stationary bicycle, that measures peak anaerobic power and anaerobic capacity. The test, which can also be performed on an arm crank ergometer, consists of a set time pedalling at maximum speed against a given resistance. The prototype test based on the Cumming's test was introduced in 1974, at the Wingate Institute and has undergone modifications as time has progressed. The Wingate test has also been used as a basis to design newer tests in the same vein, and others that use running as the exercise instead of cycling. Sprint interval testing such as is similar to the construction of the Wingate test has been shown to increase both aerobic and anaerobic performance.

The Wingate Test was developed at the Wingate Institute in Israel during the 1970s.

Validity

To determine testing procedure validity, one must test the protocol against a "gold standard" trusted to elicit "true" values. In instances where there is such a standard, such as hydrostatic weighing to determine body composition, this is easy. There is however no such standard protocol for the determination of either anaerobic capacity or power, due to this problem, the Wingate test has instead been compared with sport performance, sport specialty, and laboratory findings. These comparisons have determined that the Wingate test is measuring what it claims to measure, and is a good indicator of these measurements. Other references question the validity because the usual method of calculating the resistance of a brake band loaded with weights does not take into account all aspects of rope-brake theory and overestimates the actual force by 12-15%.

Application

The Wingate test is believed to show two things: all-out peak anaerobic power and anaerobic capacity. These two values have been reported as important factors in sports with quick, all-out efforts. Short sprinting events rely heavily upon the anaerobic energy pathways during execution, which leads to speculation that greater performance in a Wingate test can predict success in these events. This has not been proven, and the more applicable theory would be that improvements in Wingate scores could predict improvements in sprinting times.

Variations

The Wingate test has undergone many variations since its inception in the 1970s. Many researchers have used a 30-sec Wingate, while others have lengthened the duration to 60-sec or even 120-sec. The main purpose of this alteration is to more fully stress both the alactic and lactic anaerobic energy systems, which are the main source of energy for the first two minutes of exercise.

Another alteration that has been made is the repetition of Wingate tests. In current literature, this test has been repeated four, five, or even six times in one testing session. Repeating the Wingate test during training sessions can increase aerobic power and capacity, as well as maximal aerobic capacity.

The last common alteration is the workload during the test. The original Wingate test used a load of 0.075 kp per kg bodyweight of the subject. As these were young subjects, some suggest that adult subjects should use higher workloads, and several different loads have been used. Katch et al. used workloads of 0.053, 0.067, and 0.080 kp per kg bodyweight, while other researchers have increased the workload even higher, to 0.098 kp per kg bodyweight. The advantage of increasing the workload can show an increased, and therefore more representative, value for peak power in collegiate athletes. The workload can be altered, but a standard Wingate test still uses the original workload.

Common Testing Procedure

Before the subject starts the Wingate test, they typically perform a low-resistance warm-up for at least five minutes to help minimize the risk of injury. During the warm-up the subject generally completes two or three 15 second "sprints" to make sure they are used to the fast movement before the test begins. On completing the warm-up the subject should rest for one minute, after which the test begins. The subject gets a five-second countdown to the beginning of the test, during which time they pedal as fast as they can. On the start of the test, the workload drops instantly (within three seconds if using a mechanical ergometer) and the subject continues to pedal quickly for 30 seconds.

An ergometer with an electromagnetic brake generally collects and displays data through a computer. With a mechanical ergometer, the researcher must count and record the number of revolutions pedaled for every five second interval during the test, and then determine power data. On test completion, the subject should pedal against low resistance in a cool-down phase.

The Wingate test can be completed on several types of bicycle ergometers, which can be controlled with either mechanical or electromagnetic brakes. If an ergometer with an electromagnetic braking system is used, it must be capable of applying a constant resistance. The most commonly used testing ergometer in the World is the Monark 894E Wingate testing ergometer.

Relevant Calculations

Peak Power (PP)

Ideally measured within the first 5 sec of the test, and is calculated by:

$$P = \frac{F \times d}{t}$$

where t is time in seconds. On an ergometer with mechanical brakes the force is the resistance (kg) added to the flywheel, while distance is:

$$d = revolutions \times d_f$$

where d_f is the distance around the flywheel (measured in meters). Peak power values are given on a computer with electromagnetically braked ergometers. Power is expressed in Watts (W).

Relative Peak Power (RPP)

This allows for comparisons between people of varying sizes and body masses, and is calculated by:

$$RPP = \frac{PP}{BW}$$

where BW is body weight.

Anaerobic Fatigue (AF)

Anaerobic fatigue shows the percentage of power lost from the beginning to end of the Wingate. This is calculated by:

$$AF = \frac{PP - LP}{PP}$$

here PP is peak power and LP is lowest power.

Anaerobic Capacity (AC)

Anaerobic capacity is the total work completed during the test duration.

$\sum_{i=0}^{n} P_i$ where P_i is power at any point starting at the beginning of the test (i) to the end (n).

Testing Considerations

Diurnal variations occur within the body in many forms, such as hormone levels and motor coordination, therefore it is important to consideration what effects may become apparent in Wingate testing. Recent studies have confirmed that circadian rhythms can significantly alter peak power output during a Wingate test. According to these studies, an early morning Wingate test elicits significantly lower peak power values than a late afternoon or evening Wingate test.

As in every physical exertion, several outside factors can play a role in Wingate performance. Motivation is present in almost every sporting event, and some believe that it can improve performance. Cognitive motivation has not been shown to influence Wingate performance; emotional motivation however has been found to improve peak power ratings. It is therefore suggested that all outside factors that involve emotion be standardized if possible in Wingate testing environments.

Another important outside factor is warm-up. According to some literature, a 15-minute intermittent warm-up improved mean power output by 7% while having no impact on peak values. These findings suggest that warm-up is an unimportant factor in peak power levels, but if mean power is the variable of interest it is important to standardize the warm-up.

Since the Wingate test stresses the anaerobic metabolic systems glucose consumption pre-testing can be another influential factor. The anaerobic energy systems use glucose as the primary energy source, and greater available glucose could influence the power output over short intervals. Therefore, glucose consumption prior to testing should be standardized between all participants.

Sampling rate can severely impact the values obtained for peak and average power output. Sampling rates consistent with a standard mechanical ergometer test show significantly lower peak and average power values than a test with much higher sampling rates in the computer data feeds. Furthermore, tests that use low sampling rates (< 2 Hz) tend to be less consistent than tests with high sampling rates. This suggests that a sampling rate of at least 5 Hz (0.2 sec) provides the most accurate results.

Other Uses

The Wingate test can also be used in training instances, especially in cyclists. In many races, cyclists finish the race with a sprint. This maximal exertion stresses anaerobic energy pathways. As Hazell et al. have demonstrated, training in this manner can increase aerobic and anaerobic performance. Since this method can increase anaerobic performance, many cycling athletes have taken to using repeated sprint intervals, such as the Wingate test, as training devices to increase performance in the final leg of the race. These Wingate tests may be slightly modified version of the standard test laid out above.

Sprinting

Sprint training is an exercise regimen that burns fat, builds muscle, and boosts BMR (Basal Metabolic Rate). Because studies have shown that short bursts of running are more efficient than long walks or jogs, sprint training is becoming the recommended method of choice for cardiovascular exercise.

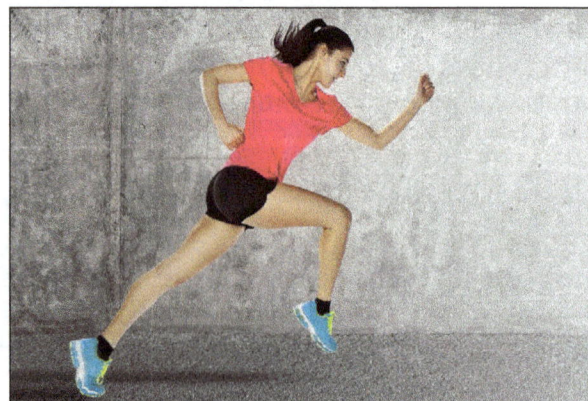

With sprint training, there are two basic ways to achieve ideal results:

- Flat sprints

- Incline sprints

What are Flat Sprints?

Flat-sprints are the perfect way for a beginner to start with sprint training. To perform flat sprints you will run at high speeds on a flat surface. For example, you might sprint on:

- A running track

- A sports field

- A jogging path

- A sidewalk in your neighbourhood

What are Incline Sprints?

Incline sprints are more advanced and require more muscle to complete without risk of injury. If you are a beginner, it is recommended that you start with flat sprints before moving up to incline sprints. To perform incline sprints, choose a hill with a steep grade and at least 50 yards of running space. For example, you might choose:

- A city park

- A hilly road

- A mountain path

How to do Sprint Training

Whether you choose to flat sprint or incline sprint, the method in which you perform sprint training is the same. To get started with sprint training, you will need:

- A stopwatch

- A good pair of running shoes or cross trainers

- Appropriate exercise attire

- Drinking water

When you have decided on a location, warm up by speed walking or jogging for about three minutes on your chosen route. If you are an incline sprinter, you can jog in place for three minutes before doing some dynamic stretches. Then, start sprinting uphill.

Your sprint time will be determined by how long you have been sprint training. Beginners usually sprint in 30-second increments. Seasoned sprinters usually sprint for 180 seconds (two and a half minutes per sprint).

Each burst of sprinting is followed by a rest period. The rest period is not for standing around or sitting, but rather for walking back to your starting spot (so you can get ready to sprint again). The constant movement helps you avoid muscle cramps while your body continues to burn calories.

References

- Rippetoe M, Kilgore L (2005). "Squat". Starting Strength. The Aasgard Company. Pp. 46–49. ISBN 978-0-9768054-0-3

- Anaerobic-exercise: verywellfit.com, Retrieved 29 March, 2019

- "How To Get Stronger: The Simple Science of Strength". What They Never Taught You In School. Retrieved 10 December 2019.

- Anaerobic-exercise-benefits, fitness-and-exercise, lifestyle, menstrual-cycle: flo.health, Retrieved 30 April, 2019

- Shaw I, Shaw BS (2014). "Resistance Training and the Prevention of Sports Injuries". In Hopkins G (ed.). Sports Injuries: Prevention, Management and Risk Factors. Hauppauge, NY: Nova Science Publishers. ISBN 9781634633055

- What-is-sprint-training, health: dummies.com, Retrieved 29 June, 2019

- "Is Training To Failure Necessary?". Training Science. 2012-03-27. Archived from the original on 2017-04-01. Retrieved 2017-03-31

5

Effects of Exercise

There are many effects of exercise which can be categorized into positive and negative effects. Some of its positive effects are improvement in agility, flexibility and physical fitness. A few of its negative effects include muscle soreness, hyponatremia, muscle cramps, etc. This chapter discusses in detail these positive and negative effects of exercise.

Physiological Effects of Exercise

The physiological response to exercise is dependent on the intensity, duration and frequency of the exercise as well as the environmental conditions. During physical exercise, requirements for oxygen and substrate in skeletal muscle are increased, as are the removal of metabolites and carbon dioxide. Chemical, mechanical and thermal stimuli affect alterations in metabolic, cardiovascular and ventilatory function in order to meet these increased demands.

Immediate Energy Sources

Adenosine Triphosphate

Adenosine triphosphate (ATP) is the common chemical intermediate that provides energy for all forms of biological work and is essential for muscle contraction. Some enzymes (ATPase) are able to use the energy stored in the bond between adenosine diphosphate (ADP) and inorganic phosphate (P_i). As water is involved this is called hydrolysis.

$$ATP + H_2O \rightarrow ADP + P_i + Energy$$

Each mole of ATP releases 7.3 kcal (30.7 kJ), and a small amount of ATP is stored in the muscle. If enough ATP was stored to fuel daily resting metabolism, it would amount to more than half of an individual's body mass. Therefore, it is essential that ATP can be resynthesized rapidly from energy-dense molecules, and, at rest, the ATP requirement of muscles is readily supplied from the oxidative metabolism of glucose and fatty acids. However, at the onset of exercise there is an immediate requirement for increased supply of energy and there is only enough ATP stored for 1–2 seconds of work and therefore rapid ways to resynthesize ATP are required.

The Adenylate Kinase Reaction

One alternative source is the adenylate kinase reaction, which results in ATP production from the conversion of two molecules of adenosine diphosphate (ADP) to adenosine monophosphate (AMP) and ATP. However, of greater quantitative importance is the utilization of phosphocreatine stored in the muscle.

Phosphocreatine System

Phosphocreatine (PCr) is another high-energy compound containing a high-energy phosphate bond that can be hydrolysed to provide energy and resynthesize ATP:

$$PCr + ADP \rightarrow ATP + PCr$$

Creatine kinase

Skeletal muscle stores of PCr provide quantitatively the greatest contribution to energy provision in the first 10 s of high intensity activities such as sprinting. PCr stores are rapidly depleted but they provide an important buffer in the first few seconds of exercise before other aspects of metabolism are activated.

Resynthesis of ATP from Energy-dense Substrates

Glycolysis

Glycolysis is the pathway by which glycogen and glucose are converted to two pyruvate molecules. In the presence of oxygen, pyruvate enters the Krebs cycle via acetyl CoA. Each turn of the Krebs cycle produces hydrogen carriers that enter the electron transport chain (ETC) and ultimately donate H^+ to oxygen to form water, allowing the ETC to proceed. However, when oxygen is not present, the ETC cannot proceed which prevents flux through the Krebs cycle and results in a build up of pyruvate. If this was allowed to continue then glycolysis would stop and no further ATP would be resynthesized. Fortunately, pyruvate can accept the hydrogen carrier, forming lactic acid via lactate dehydrogenase (LDH). The conversion of glycogen to lactic acid yields only 3 mol ATP per molecule of glycogen, but this can occur in the absence of oxygen and the maximum rate of glycolysis can be reached within a few seconds of the onset of exercise. In contrast, complete breakdown of glycogen via glycolysis, the Krebs cycle and the ETC yields 39 ATP per molecule of glycogen.

Fat metabolism

Fatty acids are more energy dense than glycogen and there are very large stores of fat in adipose tissue. In fact, if all of the energy stored as fat were stored as glycogen, body mass would increase by ~50 kg. Fatty acids are catabolized via β-oxidation and then entry to the Krebs cycle and the ETC. If it is fully oxidized a typical fat (palmitate) yields 129 molecules of ATP. Given that stores of fat in the body are so vast, they would allow exercise at a maximal intensity (i.e. sprinting) to continue for >1 h. However, the rate of ATP resynthesis from fat is too slow to be of great importance during high intensity activity. Therefore, although fat is the preferred substrate and dominates the energy contribution to resting metabolism, carbohydrate stores are available when energy requirements increase, for example at the onset of exercise. As exercise continues, however, fat metabolism may become more important, particularly if muscle glycogen stores become depleted.

Traditionally, protein is not considered to contribute to energy provision except under conditions of starvation or in ultra-endurance events. This is unsurprising on the basis that most of the protein in the body is functional in nature, for example contractile proteins in skeletal muscle.

Muscle Types

Muscle fibres can be classified as type I, type IIa and type IIb fibres. Characteristics of type I (slow twitch) and type IIb (fast twitch) fibres are summarized in Table. The proportion of type I and type II fibres varies in different muscles, with greater proportions of type I fibres in postural muscles. Type I fibres are more suited to prolonged activity as they are more efficient than type II fibres and have a greater reliance on oxidative metabolism of fatty acids and glycogen. Therefore, during prolonged, low intensity activity, type I fibres will be recruited. However, as the force required increases, larger type II fibres are recruited. If the speed of contraction is rapid, only type II fibres can contribute to force generation since type I fibres cannot produce force at as fast a rate as type II fibres. There are hereditary differences in the proportion of each type of fibre in a given muscle, which determine to some degree the athletic capabilities of the individual. For example, some people appear to be more suited to marathon running (type I predominant) whereas others are born to sprint and jump (type II predominant).

Table: Characteristics of Type I and II muscles.

Characteristic	Type I	Type II
Time to peak tension	~110 ms	~50 ms
Macroscopic colour	Red	White
Capillary supply	High	Low
Main energy system	Aerobic	Anaerobic
Myoglobin levels	High	Low
Number of mitochondria	High	Low
Oxidative enzymes levels	High	Low
Resistance to fatigue	Low	High
Type of exercise suited	Endurance/long-distance runner	High intensity/sprinter

Respiratory System

During exercise, ventilation might increase from resting values of around 5–6 litre min^{-1} to >100 litre min^{-1}. Ventilation increases linearly with increases in work rate at submaximal exercise intensities. Oxygen consumption also increases linearly with increasing work rate at submaximal intensities. In an average young male, resting oxygen consumption is about 250 ml min^{-1} and in an endurance athlete oxygen consumption during very high intensity exercise might reach 5000 ml min^{-1}. The increase in pulmonary ventilation is attributable to a combination of increases in tidal volume and respiratory rate and closely matches the increase in oxygen uptake and carbon dioxide output. Breathing capacity, however, does not reach its maximum even during strenuous exercise and it is not responsible for the limitation in oxygen delivery to muscles seen during high intensity activity. Haemoglobin continues to be fully saturated with oxygen throughout exercise in people with normal respiratory function.

Changes in Arterial Blood Gases

The changes which occur in arterial pH, PO_2 and PCO_2 values during exercise are usually small. Arterial PO_2 often rises slightly because of hyperventilation although it may eventually fall at high work rates. During vigorous exercise, when sufficient oxygen for flux through the Krebs cycle is not available, the increased reliance on glycolysis results in increased accumulation of lactic acid, which initially leads to an increase in $PaCO_2$. However, this is counteracted by the stimulation of ventilation and as a result $PaCO_2$ is decreased. This provides some respiratory compensation for further lactic acid production and prevents a decline in blood pH, which remains nearly constant during moderate exercise.

Changes in Ventilation

Ventilation increases abruptly in the initial stages of exercise and is then followed by a more gradual increase. The rapid rise in ventilation at the onset of exercise is thought to be attributable to motor centre activity and afferent impulses from proprioceptors of the limbs, joints and muscles. The mechanism of stimulation following this first stage is not completely understood. Arterial oxygen and carbon dioxide tensions are not sufficiently abnormal to stimulate respiration during exercise. Suggestions have been made that the sensitivity of peripheral chemoreceptors to oscillations in PaO_2 and $PaCO_2$ is responsible for increasing ventilation, even though the absolute values remain stable. Central chemoreceptors may be readjusted to increase ventilation to maintain carbon dioxide concentrations. Other theories are that the rise in body temperature may play a role, or that collateral branches of neurogenic impulses from the motor cortex to active muscles and joints may stimulate the brain stem and respiratory centre leading to hyperpnoea. Overall, a number of factors have been suggested for the increase in ventilation, which occurs with exercise. The respiratory rate might remain elevated after heavy exercise for up to 1–2 h.

Cardiovascular System

Substrate and oxygen requirements of working skeletal muscles are dramatically elevated above resting requirements. Resting blood flow to muscle is usually 2–4 ml·100 g muscle^{-1} min^{-1}, but might increase to nearly 100 ml·100 g muscle^{-1} min^{-1} during maximal exercise. This occurs in part because of vasodilatory metabolites such as AMP, adenosine, H^+, K^+ and PO_3^{-4}, PO_4^{3-} acting on pre-capillary sphincters, which override the vasoconstrictor effects of norepinephrine. In addition, decreased pH and increased temperature shift the oxygen dissociation curve for haemoglobin to the right in exercising muscle. This assists in unloading more oxygen from the blood into the muscle. During muscular contraction, blood flow is restricted briefly but overall it is enhanced by the pumping action of the muscle.

Whilst muscle and coronary blood flow increase, cerebral blood flow is maintained constant and splanchnic flow diminishes. However, essential organs such as the bowel and kidneys must be protected with some blood flow maintained. An additional demand on blood flow during exercise is the requirement to increase skin blood flow in order to enable heat dissipation.

Circulatory Changes

The increase in blood flow to muscles requires an increase in the cardiac output, which is in direct proportion to the increase in oxygen consumption. The cardiac output is increased by both a rise in the heart rate and the stroke volume attributable to a more complete emptying of the heart by a forcible systolic contraction. These chronotropic and inotropic effects on the heart are brought about by stimulation from the noradrenergic sympathetic nervous system. The increase in heart rate is also mediated by vagal inhibition and is sustained by autonomic sympathetic responses and carbon dioxide acting on the medulla.

The efficacy of systolic contraction is particularly important in trained athletes who can achieve significant increases in cardiac output as a consequence of hypertrophy of cardiac muscle. Table shows that increased maximal cardiac output in endurance trained athletes is a function of greater stroke volume rather than an increase in maximal heart rate, which is, in fact, lower in these athletes.

Comparison of cardiac function between athletes and non-athletes.

	Stroke volume (ml)	Heart rate (beats min^{-1})
At rest		
Non-athlete	70	70
Trained athlete	100	50
Maximum exercise		
Non-athlete	110	190
Trained athlete	160	180

Heart rate and stroke volume increase to about 90% of their maximum values during strenuous exercise and cardiovascular function is the limiting factor for oxygen delivery to the tissues. Oxygen utilization by the body can never be more than the rate at which the cardiovascular system can transport oxygen to the tissues. There is only a moderate increase in blood pressure secondary to the rise in cardiac output. This is caused by stretching of the walls of the arterioles and vasodilatation, which in combination reduce overall peripheral vascular resistance. There is a large increase in venous return as a consequence of muscular contraction, blood diversion from the viscera and vasoconstriction.

Maximum Oxygen Consumption

As work rate is increased, oxygen uptake increases linearly. However, there is an upper limit to oxygen uptake and, therefore, above a certain work rate oxygen consumption reaches a plateau. This is termed the maximal oxygen uptake $\dot{V}\text{co}_{2\,max}$. A considerable amount of research has focused on the factors that limit $\dot{V}\text{co}_{2\,max}$.

The Pulmonary System

Pulmonary limitations to $\dot{V}\text{co}_{2\,max}$ are evident in some situations, such as when exercising at high altitudes and in individuals with asthma or other types of chronic obstructive pulmonary disease. However, in most individuals exercising at sea level the lungs perform their role of saturating arterial blood with oxygen extremely effectively as described previously.

Cardiac Output

As described previously, endurance training results in increased cardiac output through increased stroke volume. This is considered to be a very important factor determining $\dot{V}O_{2\,max}$ in the normal range of $\dot{V}O_{2\,max}$ values. In addition, β-blockade reduces cardiac output and results in a concomitant reduction in $\dot{V}O_{2\,max}$. During maximal exercise, almost all of the available oxygen in the blood is extracted by skeletal muscle, and for this reason it appears that delivery of oxygen through increased blood flow is the most important factor limiting $\dot{V}O_{2\,max}$.

Oxygen Carrying Capacity of the Blood

A reduction in the oxygen carrying capacity in conditions such as anaemia produces fatigue and shortness of breath on mild exertion. Some athletes have tried to increase red blood cell levels by removing, storing and then reinfusing them. This method of 'blood doping' has been shown to improve $\dot{V}O_{2\,max}$ by up to 10%. More recently, there has been evidence of erythropoietin abuse in sport in order to increase red blood cell levels. The improvements in $\dot{V}O_{2\,max}$ observed when employing these methods provide good evidence that oxygen delivery is a limiting factor for $\dot{V}O_{2\,max}$.

Skeletal Muscle Limitations

The factors listed above can be considered as 'central' factors in the same way that potential limitations in the skeletal muscle are considered 'peripheral' factors limiting $\dot{V}O_{2\,max}$.

Peripheral factors include properties of skeletal muscle such as levels of mitochondrial enzymes and capillary density. As mitochondria are the sites of oxygen consumption (in the final stage of the ETC), doubling the number of mitochondria should double oxygen uptake in the muscle. However, this is not the case, suggesting that the number of mitochondria are not limiting to $\dot{V}O_{2\,max}$.

Capillary density is known to increase with endurance training, with the effect of increasing transit time of blood through the muscle, and improving oxygen extraction from the muscle. It has been suggested that there is a relationship between capillary density and $\dot{V}O_{2\,max}$.

In summary, a reduction in any of the factors involved in the delivery and utilization of oxygen will decrease $\dot{V}O_{2\,max}$.

However, in healthy individuals carrying out whole-body maximal exercise at sea level, the ability of the cardiorespiratory system to deliver oxygen to the working muscles rather than the ability of the muscles to consume the oxygen is limiting.

Body Temperature

The maximum efficiency for the conversion of energy nutrients into muscular work is 20–25%. The remainder is released in a non-usable form as heat energy, which raises the body temperature. In order to dissipate the extra heat generated as a result of increased metabolism during exercise, blood supply to the skin must be increased. This is achieved with vasodilatation of cutaneous vessels by inhibition of the vasoconstrictor tone. Evaporation of sweat is also a major pathway for heat loss and further heat is lost in the expired air with ventilation.

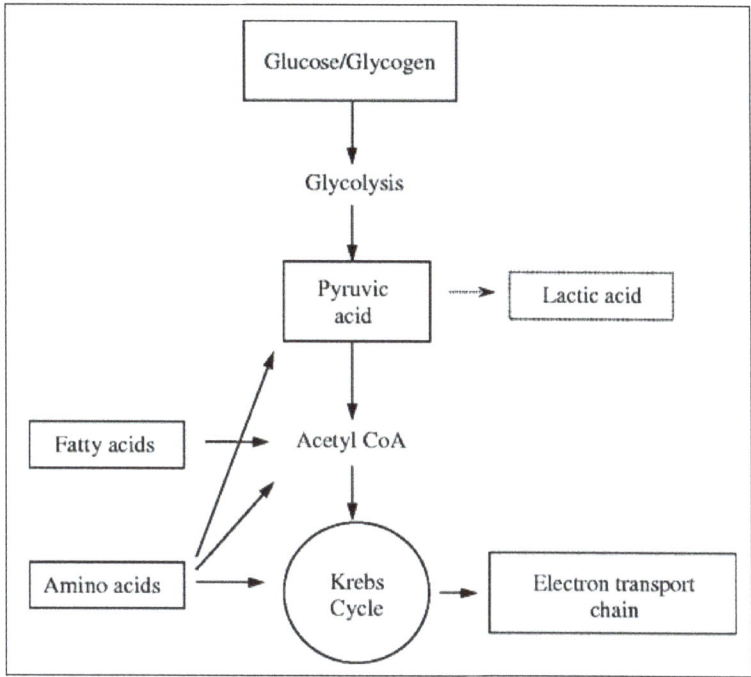

An overview of substrate metabolism.

The hypothalamus is responsible for thermoregulation and it is important that this process is effective. However, during exercise in hot, humid conditions evaporative heat loss through sweating might not be able to remove sufficient heat from the body. Regulation of body temperature may fail and temperatures may be high enough to cause heat stroke. This presents with symptoms of extreme weakness, exhaustion, headache, dizziness eventually leading to collapse and unconsciousness.

Positive Effects

Agility

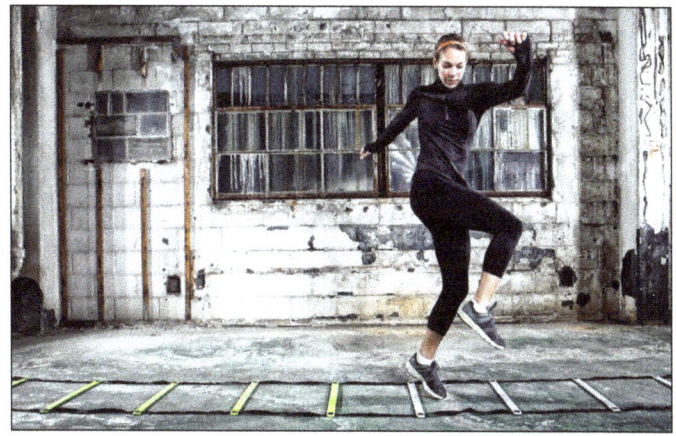

Agility is the ability to move and change direction and position of the body quickly and effectively while under control. It requires quick reflexes, coordination, balance, speed, and correct response to the changing situation.

To be agile, you are responding to what is going on around you, taking in that information and translating it into body positioning that will maintain balance and control. You are moving to the best position to take the next action, such as catching a ball or making a tackle. You are moving in a way that your body and sports equipment are in the right position to take the next action effectively.

Agility as a Key Component of Sports and Physical Activities

Agility is one of the key components of fitness and is valuable in many sports and physical activities. Think of the sports where you have to use agility. In team sports such as football, soccer, basketball, hockey, volleyball and rugby you must quickly respond to movements of the other players and of the ball.

In tennis, handball, squash, table tennis and similar individual sports, you have to quickly respond to the position of the ball. In surfing, skiing and snowboarding you must be agile to respond to the changing conditions of the surface of the water and snow.

Agility Tests

Shuttle runs are often done as an agility test as well as a drill to build sports agility. Markers are set up and you sprint from one marker to the other, do a quick turn and sprint back. The U.S. Military Academy uses a shuttle run test. The National Football League uses a 5-10-5 shuttle run as an agility test and drill.

The SPARQ rating combines testing for speed, power, agility, reaction and quickness. It is sport-specific as well as a test for general athleticism. The general assessment tests include the agility shuttle 5-10-5 to measure agility. For sport-specific agility, they use a lane agility drill for basketball, a shuttle cross pick-up for hockey, and the arrowhead drill for soccer. The SPARQ rating is used by many sports training companies and certified SPARQ trainers.

Agility Drills for Athletes

A variety of agility drills can be used in different sports to develop speed and coordination.

- Lateral plyometric jumps: Jumps made to the side.

- Tuck jumps: Jumping straight up from a squat position, remaining tucked at the top of the jump before extending your legs to land.

- Shuttle runs: Sprinting from marker to marker with frequent changes in direction.

- Forward-backward sprints: Sprint forward to a cone, then jog backward to the start.

- Speed Ladder Agility Drills: These use a piece of equipment that looks like a ladder, and drills can be done running forward with high knees to improve foot speed for field sports, or running laterally to improve agility for court sports.

- Dot Drills: These use an X-shaped pattern to jump from dot to dot with both feet at the same time. It is used for field and racket sports as well as skiing and basketball.

Physical Fitness

Physical fitness is a state of health and well-being and, more specifically, the ability to perform aspects of sports, occupations and daily activities. Physical fitness is generally achieved through proper nutrition, moderate-vigorous physical exercise, and sufficient rest.

Before the industrial revolution, *fitness* was defined as the capacity to carry out the day's activities without undue fatigue. However, with automation and changes in lifestyles *physical fitness* is now considered a measure of the body's ability to function efficiently and effectively in work and leisure activities, to be healthy, to resist hypokinetic diseases, and to meet emergency situations.

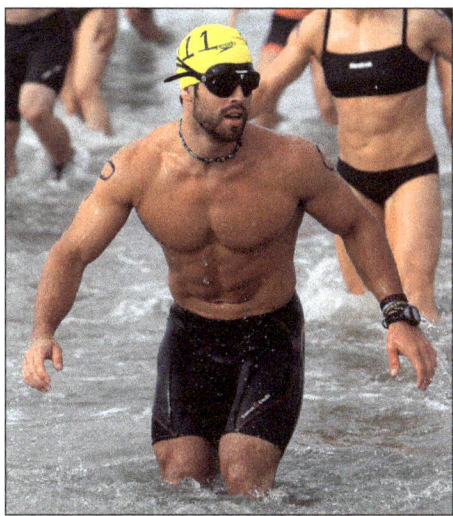

Physical fitness is generally achieved through exercise. Photo shows
Rich Froning Jr. – four-time winner of "Fittest Man on Earth" title.

Fitness

Fitness is defined as the quality or state of being fit. Around 1950, perhaps consistent with the Industrial Revolution and the treatise of World War II, the term "fitness" increased in western vernacular by a factor of ten. The modern definition of fitness describes either a person or machine's ability to perform a specific function or a holistic definition of human adaptability to cope with various situations. This has led to an interrelation of human fitness and attractiveness that has mobilized global fitness and fitness equipment industries. Regarding specific function, fitness is attributed to persons who possess significant aerobic or anaerobic ability, i.e. endurance or strength. A well-rounded fitness program improves a person in all aspects of fitness compared to practicing only one, such as only cardio/respiratory endurance or only weight training.

A comprehensive fitness program tailored to an individual typically focuses on one or more specific skills, and on age- or health-related needs such as bone health. Many sources also cite mental, social and emotional health as an important part of overall fitness. This is often presented in textbooks as a triangle made up of three points, which represent physical, emotional, and mental fitness. Physical fitness can also prevent or treat many chronic health conditions brought on by unhealthy lifestyle or aging. Working out can also help some people sleep better and possibly alleviate some mood disorders in certain individuals.

Developing research has demonstrated that many of the benefits of exercise are mediated through the role of skeletal muscle as an endocrine organ. That is, contracting muscles release multiple substances known as myokines, which promote the growth of new tissue, tissue repair, and various anti-inflammatory functions, which in turn reduce the risk of developing various inflammatory diseases.

Training

Specific or task-oriented fitness is a person's ability to perform in a specific activity with a reasonable efficiency: for example, sports or military service. Specific training prepares athletes to perform well in their sport.

Examples are:

- 100 m sprint: in a sprint, the athlete must be trained to work anaerobically throughout the race, an example of how to do this would be interval training.

- Century Ride: cyclists must be prepared aerobically for a bike ride of 100 miles or more.

- Middle distance running: athletes require both speed and endurance to gain benefit out of this training. The hard-working muscles are at their peak for a longer period of time as they are being used at that level for the longer period of time.

- Marathon: in this case, the athlete must be trained to work aerobically and their endurance must be built-up to a maximum.

- Many firefighters and police officers undergo regular fitness testing to determine if they are capable of the physically demanding tasks required of the job.

- Members of armed forces are often required to pass a formal fitness test. For example, soldiers of the US Army must be able to pass the Army Physical Fitness Test (APFT).

- Hill sprints: requires a level of fitness to begin with; the exercise is particularly good for the leg muscles. The army often trains to do mountain climbing and races.

- Plyometric and isometric exercises: an excellent way to build strength and increase muscular endurance.

- Sand running creates less strain on leg muscles than running on grass or concrete. This is because sand collapses beneath the foot, softening the landing. Sand training is an effective way to lose weight and become fit, as more effort is needed (one and a half times more) to run on the soft sand than on a hard surface.

- Aquajogging is a form of exercise that decreases strain on joints and bones. The water supplies minimal impact to muscles and bones, which is good for those recovering from injury. Furthermore, the resistance of the water as one jogs through it provides an enhanced effect of exercise (the deeper you are the greater the force needed to pull your leg through).

- Swimming: Squatting exercise helps in enhancing a swimmer's start.

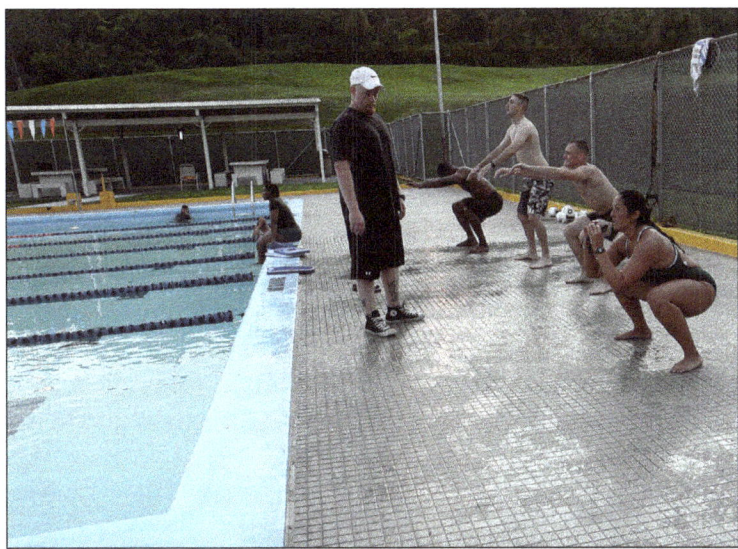
Swimmers perform squats prior to entering the pool.

For physical fitness activity to benefit an individual, the exertion triggers a response called a stimulus. Exercise with the correct amount of intensity, duration, and frequency can produce a significant amount of improvement. The person may overall feel better, but the physical effects on the human body take weeks or months to notice and possibly years for full development. For training purposes, exercise must provide a stress or demand on either a function or tissue. To continue improvements, this demand must eventually increase little over an extended period of time. This sort of exercise training has three basic principles: overload, specificity, and progression. These principles are related to health but also enhancement of physical working capacity.

High Intensity Interval Training

High intensity interval training (HIIT) consists of repeated, short bursts of exercise, completed at a high level of intensity. These sets of intense activity are followed by a predetermined time of rest or low intensity activity. Studies have shown that exercising at a higher intensity has increased cardiac benefits for humans, compared to when exercising at a low or moderate level. When your workout consists of an HIIT session, your body has to work harder to replace the oxygen it lost. Research into the benefits of HIIT have revealed that it can be very successful for reducing fat, especially around the abdominal region. Furthermore, when compared to continuous moderate exercise, HIIT proves to burn more calories and increase the amount of fat burned post- HIIT session. Lack of time is one of the main reasons stated for not exercising; HIIT is a great alternative for those people because the duration of an HIIT session can be as short as 10 minutes, making it much quicker than conventional workouts.

Effects

Controlling Blood Pressure

Physical fitness has proven to result in positive effects on the body's blood pressure because staying active and exercising regularly builds up a stronger heart. The heart is the main organ in charge of systolic blood pressure and diastolic blood pressure. Engaging in a physical activity raises blood pressure. Once the subject stops the activity, the blood pressure returns to normal. The more physical activity that one engages in, the easier this process becomes, resulting in a more 'fit' individual. Through regular physical fitness, the heart does not have to work as hard to create a rise in blood pressure, which lowers the force on the arteries, and lowers the overall blood pressure.

Cancer Prevention

Centers for disease control and prevention provide lifestyle guidelines of maintaining a balanced diet and engaging in physical activity to reduce the risk of disease. The WCRF/ American Institute for Cancer Research (AICR) published a list of recommendations that reflect the evidence they have found through consistency in fitness and dietary factors that directly relate to cancer prevention.

The WCRF/AICR recommendations include the following:

- Be as lean as possible without becoming underweight.

- Each week, adults should engage in at least 150 minutes of moderate intensity physical activity or 75 minutes of vigorous intensity physical activity.

- Children should engage in at least one hour of moderate or vigorous physical activity each week.

- Be physically active for at least thirty minutes every day.

- Avoid sugar, and limit the consumption of energy packed foods.

- Balance one's diet with a variety of vegetables, grains, fruits, legumes, etc.

- Limit sodium intake, the consumption of red meats and the consumption of processed meats.

- Limit alcoholic drinks to two for men and one for women a day.

These recommendations are also widely supported by the American Cancer Society. The guidelines have been evaluated and individuals that have higher guideline adherence scores substantially reduce cancer risk as well as help towards control with a multitude of chronic health problems. Regular physical activity is a factor that helps reduce an individual's blood pressure and improves cholesterol levels, two key components that correlate with heart disease and Type 2 Diabetes. The American Cancer Society encourages the public to "adopt a physically active lifestyle" by meeting the criteria in a variety of physical activities such as hiking, swimming, circuit training, resistance training, lifting, etc. It is understood that cancer is not a disease that can be cured by physical fitness alone, however, because it is a multifactorial disease, physical fitness is a controllable prevention. The large associations tied with being physically fit and reduced cancer risk are enough to provide a strategy to reduce cancer risk. The American Cancer Society asserts different levels of activity ranging from moderate to vigorous to clarify the recommended time spent on a physical activity. These classifications of physical activity consider the intentional exercise and basic activities are done on a daily basis and give the public a greater understanding of what fitness levels suffice as future disease prevention.

Inflammation

Studies have shown an association between increased physical activity and reduced inflammation. It produces both a short-term inflammatory response and a long-term anti-inflammatory effect. Physical activity reduces inflammation in conjunction with or independent of changes in body weight. However, the mechanisms linking physical activity to inflammation are unknown.

Immune System

Physical activity boosts the immune system. This is dependent on the concentration of endogenous factors (such as sex hormones, metabolic hormones and growth hormones), body temperature, blood flow, hydration status and body position. Physical activity has shown to increase the levels of natural killer (NK) cells, T cells, macrophages, neutrophils and eosinophils, complements, cytokines, antibodies and T cytotoxic cells. However, the mechanism linking physical activity to immune system is not fully understood.

Weight Control

Achieving resilience through physical fitness promotes a vast and complex range of health-related benefits. Individuals who keep up physical fitness levels generally regulate their distribution of body fat and stay away from obesity. Abdominal fat, specifically visceral fat, is most directly affected by engaging in aerobic exercise. Strength training has been known to increase the amount of muscle in the body, however, it can also reduce body fat. Sex steroid hormones, insulin, and an appropriate immune response are factors that mediate metabolism in relation to the abdominal fat. Therefore, physical fitness provides weight control through regulation of these bodily functions.

Menopause and Physical Fitness

Menopause is often said to have occurred when a woman has had no vaginal bleeding for over a year since her last menstrual cycle. There are a number of symptoms connected to menopause, most of which can affect the quality of life of a woman involved in this stage of her life. One way to reduce the severity of the symptoms is to exercise and keep a healthy level of fitness. Prior to and during menopause, as the female body changes, there can be physical, physiological or internal changes to the body. These changes can be reduced or even prevented with regular exercise. These changes include:

- Preventing weight gain: around menopause women tend to experience a reduction in muscle mass and an increase in fat levels. Increasing the amount of physical exercise undertaken can help to prevent these changes.

- Reducing the risk of breast cancer: weight loss from regular exercise may offer protection from breast cancer.

- Strengthening bones: physical activity can slow the bone loss associated with menopause, reducing the chance of bone fractures and osteoporosis.

- Reducing the risk of disease: excess weight can increase the risk of heart disease and type 2 diabetes, and regular physical activity can counter these effects.

- Boosting mood: being involved in regular activities it can improve psychological health, an effect that can be seen at any age and not just during or after menopause.

The Melbourne Women's Midlife Health Project provided evidence that showed over an eight-year time period 438 were followed. Even though the physical activity was not associated with VMS in this cohort at the beginning. Women who reported they were physically active every day at the beginning were 49% less likely to have reported bothersome hot flushes. This is in contrast to women whose level of activity decreased and were more likely to experience bothersome hot flushes.

Mental Health

Studies have shown that physical activity can improve mental health and well-being. This improvement is due to an increase in blood flow to the brain and the release of hormones. Being physically fit and working out on a consistent and constant basis can positively impact one's mental health and bring about several other benefits, such as the following:

- Physical activity has been linked to the alleviation of depression and anxiety symptoms.

- In patients suffering from schizophrenia, physical fitness has been shown to improve their quality of life and decrease the effects of schizophrenia.

- Being fit can improve one's self-esteem.

- Working out can improve one's mental alertness and it can reduce fatigue.

- Studies have shown a reduction in stress levels.

- Increased opportunity for social interaction, allowing for improved social skills.

To achieve some of these benefits, the Centers for Disease Control and Prevention suggests at least 30–60 minutes of exercise 3-5 times a week.

Muscle Hypertrophy

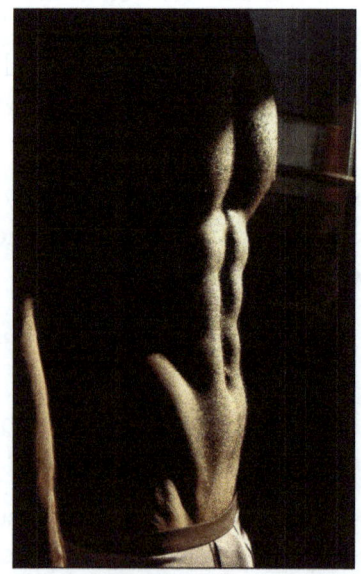

Athletes use a combination of strength training, diet, and nutritional supplementation to induce muscle hypertrophy.

Muscle hypertrophy involves an increase in size of skeletal muscle through a growth in size of its component cells. Two factors contribute to hypertrophy: sarcoplasmic hypertrophy, which focuses more on increased muscle glycogen storage; and myofibrillar hypertrophy, which focuses more on increased myofibril size.

Hypertrophy Stimulation

A range of stimuli can increase the volume of muscle cells. These changes occur as an adaptive response that serves to increase the ability to generate force or resist fatigue in anaerobic conditions.

Strength Training

Strength training, or resistance exercise, brings about neural and muscular adaptations which increase the capacity of an athlete to exert force through voluntary muscular contraction. After an initial period, in which neuro-muscular adaptation dominates, a process of muscular hypertrophy is observed whereby the size of muscle tissue increases. This increase in size is due to growth from adding sarcomeres (contractile elements) as well as an increase in non-contractile elements like sarcoplasmic fluid. The precise mechanisms which induce muscular hypertrophy are not clearly understood, with currently accepted hypotheses regarding some combination of mechanical tension, metabolic fatigue, and muscular damage as relevant factors. Progressive overload, a strategy of progressively increasing resistance or repetitions over successive bouts of exercise in order to maintain a high level of effort, is one fundamental principle of training strongly associated with muscular hypertrophy. Across the research literature, a wide variety of resistance exercise training modalities have all been shown to elicit similar hypertrophic responses in muscle tissue. Muscular hypertrophy plays an important role in competitive bodybuilding as well as strength sports like powerlifting, football and Olympic weightlifting.

Anaerobic Training

The best approach to specifically achieve muscle growth remains controversial (as opposed to focusing on gaining strength, power, or endurance); it was generally considered that consistent anaerobic strength training will produce hypertrophy over the long term, in addition to its effects on muscular strength and endurance. Muscular hypertrophy can be increased through strength training and other short-duration, high-intensity anaerobic exercises. Lower-intensity, longer-duration aerobic exercise generally does not result in very effective tissue hypertrophy; instead, endurance athletes enhance storage of fats and carbohydrates within the muscles, as well as neovascularization.

Temporary Swelling

During a workout, increased blood flow to metabolically active areas causes muscles to temporarily increase in size, also known as being "pumped up" or getting "a pump". About two hours after a workout and typically for seven to eleven days, muscles swell due to an inflammation response as tissue damage is repaired. Longer-term hypertrophy occurs due to more permanent changes in muscle structure.

Factors Affecting Hypertrophy

Biological factors (such as DNA and sex), nutrition, and training variables can affect muscle hypertrophy.

Individual differences in genetics account for a substantial portion of the variance in existing muscle mass. A classical twin study design (similar to those of behavioral genetics) estimates that about 52% of the variance in lean body mass is estimated to be heritable and that about 45% of the variance in muscle fiber proportion is genetic as well.

During puberty in males, hypertrophy occurs at an increased rate. Natural hypertrophy normally stops at full growth in the late teens. As testosterone is one of the body's major growth hormones, on average, males find hypertrophy much easier (on an absolute scale) to achieve than females and on average, have about 60% more muscle mass than women. Taking additional testosterone, as in anabolic steroids, will increase results. It is also considered a performance-enhancing drug, the use of which can cause competitors to be suspended or banned from competitions. Testosterone is also a medically regulated substance in most countries, making it illegal to possess without a medical prescription. Anabolic steroid use can cause testicular atrophy, cardiac arrest, and gynecomastia.

A positive energy balance, when more calories are consumed rather than burned, is required for anabolism and therefore muscle hypertrophy. An increased requirement for protein, especially branch chained amino acids, is required for elevated protein synthesis that is seen in athletes training for muscle hypertrophy.

Training variables, in the context of strength training, such as frequency, intensity, and total volume also directly affect the increase of muscle hypertrophy. A gradual increase in all of these training variables will yield the muscular hypertrophy.

Changes in Protein Synthesis and Muscle Cell Biology Associated with Stimuli

Protein Synthesis

The message filters down to alter the pattern of gene expression. The additional contractile proteins appear to be incorporated into existing myofibrils (the chains of sarcomeres within a muscle cell). There appears to be some limit to how large a myofibril can become: at some point, they split. These events appear to occur within each muscle fiber. That is, hypertrophy results primarily from the growth of each muscle cell, rather than an increase in the number of cells. Skeletal muscle cells are however unique in the body in that they can contain multiple nuclei, and the number of nuclei can increase.

Cortisol decreases amino acid uptake by muscle tissue, and inhibits protein synthesis. The short-term increase in protein synthesis that occurs subsequent to resistance training returns to normal after approximately 28 hours in adequately fed male youths. Another study determined that muscle protein synthesis was elevated even 72 hours following training.

A small study performed on young and elderly found that ingestion of 340 grams of lean beef (90 g protein) did not increase muscle protein synthesis any more than ingestion of 113 grams of lean beef (30 g protein). In both groups, muscle protein synthesis increased by 50%. The study concluded that more than 30 g protein in a single meal did not further enhance the stimulation of muscle protein synthesis in young and elderly. However, this study didn't check protein synthesis in relation to training; therefore conclusions from this research are controversial.

It is not uncommon for bodybuilders to advise a protein intake as high as 2–4 g per kilogram of bodyweight per day. However, scientific literature has suggested this is higher than necessary, as protein intakes greater than 1.8 g per kilogram of body weight showed to have no greater effect on muscle hypertrophy. A study carried out by American College of Sports Medicine put the recommended daily protein intake for athletes at 1.2–1.8 g per kilogram of body weight. Conversely, Di Pasquale, citing recent studies, recommends a minimum protein intake of 2.2 g/kg "for anyone involved in competitive or intense recreational sports who wants to maximize lean body mass but does not wish to gain weight. However athletes involved in strength events (..) may need even more to maximize body composition and athletic performance. In those attempting to minimize body fat and thus maximize body composition, for example in sports with weight classes and in bodybuilding, it's possible that protein may well make up over 50% of their daily caloric intake."

Microtrauma

Microtrauma, which is tiny damage to the fibers, may play a significant role in muscle growth. When microtrauma occurs (from weight training or other strenuous activities), the body responds by overcompensating, replacing the damaged tissue and adding more, so that the risk of repeat damage is reduced. Damage to these fibers has been theorized as the possible cause for the symptoms of delayed onset muscle soreness (DOMS), and is why progressive overload is essential to continued improvement, as the body adapts and becomes more resistant to stress. However, work examining the time course of changes in muscle protein synthesis and their relationship to hypertrophy showed that damage was unrelated to hypertrophy. In fact, in that study the authors showed that it was not until the damage subsided that protein synthesis was directed to muscle growth.

Myofibrillar vs. Sarcoplasmic Hypertrophy

In the bodybuilding and fitness community and even in some academic books skeletal muscle hypertrophy is described as being in one of two types: Sarcoplasmic or myofibrillar. According to this hypothesis, during sarcoplasmic hypertrophy, the volume of sarcoplasmic fluid in the muscle cell increases with no accompanying increase in muscular strength, whereas during myofibrillar hypertrophy, actin and myosin contractile proteins increase in number and add to muscular strength as well as a small increase in the size of the muscle. Sarcoplasmic hypertrophy is greater in the muscles of bodybuilders because studies suggest sarcoplasmic hypertrophy shows a greater increase in muscle size while myofibrillar hypertrophy proves to increase overall muscular strength making it more dominant in Olympic weightlifters. These two forms of adaptations rarely occur completely independently of one another; one can experience a large increase in fluid with a slight increase in proteins, a large increase in proteins with a small increase in fluid, or a relatively balanced combination of the two.

Aerobic Conditioning

Aerobic conditioning is a process whereby the heart and lungs are trained to pump blood more efficiently, allowing more oxygen to be delivered to muscles and organs.

Aerobic conditioning is the use of continuous, rhythmic movement of large muscle groups to strengthen the heart and lungs (cardiovascular system). Improvement in aerobic conditioning occurs when athletes expose themselves to an increase in oxygen uptake and metabolism, but to keep this level of aerobic conditioning, the athletes must keep or progressively increase their training to increase their aerobic conditioning.

Aerobic condition is usually achieved through cardiovascular exercise such as running, swimming, aerobics, etc. A stronger heart does not pump more blood by beating faster but by beating more efficiently. Trained endurance athletes can have resting heart rates as low as the reported 28 beats per minute in people such as Miguel Indurain or 32 beats per minute of Lance Armstrong, both of whom were professional cyclists at the highest level.

Cardiovascular Conditioning

Aerobic conditioning trains the heart to be more effective at pumping blood around the body, it does this in a multitude of ways:

- Increasing the stroke volume of the heart (how much blood the heart is pumping per beat).

- Increasing the diameter of the blood vessels, which allows for more blood to be moved through the body, which in turn allows for more oxygen to be diffused into the muscle cells.

- Increasing the size of the heart chambers, enlarging the heart so it can hold and pump more blood.

Effect of Aerobic Conditioning on Maximum Oxygen Intake

Aerobic conditioning has the ability to raise a person's maximum oxygen intake, meaning that they are able to diffuse more oxygen into their blood than they previously could.

Although exercising at lower intensities will improve aerobic conditioning, the most rapid gains are made when exercising close to an individual's anaerobic threshold. This is the intensity at which the heart and lungs can no longer provide adequate oxygen to the working muscles and an oxygen debt begins to accrue; at this point the exercise becomes anaerobic. Anaerobic training intensity for most individuals will be <85-92% of maximum heart rate.

Once improvement in aerobic conditioning is apparent, for example in metabolism and oxygen uptake, the body will progressively adapt to further training. Aerobic conditioning can be anywhere from walking on the treadmill to mowing the lawn. The average healthy person should engage in 150–200 minutes of moderate aerobic exercise every week. This amount of physical activity should help with maintaining a healthy weight and keeping the cardiovascular system in good condition.

Aerobic conditioning has many advantages over anaerobic as it can increase physical endurance and lifespan. During aerobic training, the aim is to improve the blood flow to the lungs, heart, and blood vessels. This particular type of training targets large muscle groups so that as the intensity of physical activity is increased, overall fitness is improved. There are many benefits to aerobic training, and the outcomes can be very rewarding. Aerobic conditioning can increase the duration that one can endure physical activity. This type of conditioning can help with heart disease, diabetes, or anxiety. Aerobic conditioning also has many non-medical benefits, such as improving mood, alleviating fatigue and stabilizing sleeping patterns. This overall type of conditioning has the most longevity to its practice and can improve a person's health and general well being immensely.

Flexibility

Flexibility or limberness refers to the range of movement in a joint or series of joints, and length in muscles that cross the joints to induce a bending movement or motion. Flexibility varies between individuals, particularly in terms of differences in muscle length of multi-joint muscles. Flexibility in some joints can be increased to a certain degree by exercise, with stretching a common exercise component to maintain or improve flexibility.

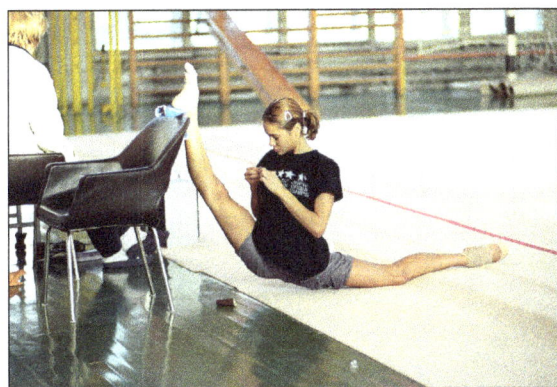

An oversplit by former Olympic gymnast Irina Tchachina.

Quality of life is enhanced by improving and maintaining a good range of motion in the joints. Overall flexibility should be developed with specific joint range of motion needs in mind as the individual joints vary from one to another. Loss of flexibility can be a predisposing factor for physical issues such as pain syndromes or balance disorders.

Sex, age, and genetics are important for range of motion. Exercise including stretching and yoga often improves flexibility.

Many factors are taken into account when establishing personal flexibility: joint structure, ligaments, tendons, muscles, skin, tissue injury, fat (or adipose) tissue, body temperature, activity level, age and sex all influence an individual's range of motion about a joint. Individual body flexibility level is measured and calculated by performing a sit and reach test, where the result is defined as personal flexibility score.

Anatomical Elements of Flexibility

Joints

The joints in a human body are surrounded by synovial membranes and articular cartilage which cover, cushion and nourish the joint and surfaces of each . Increasing muscular elasticity of the joint's range of mobility increases flexibility.

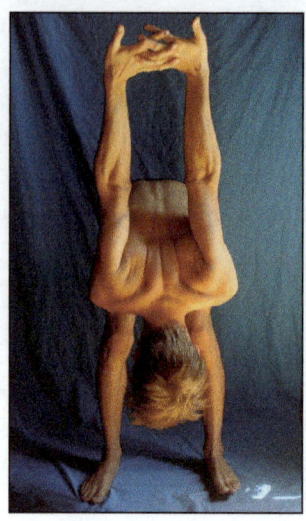
Man stretching.

Ligaments

Ligaments are composed of two different tissues: white and yellow. The white fibrous tissues are not stretchy, but are extremely strong so that even if the bone were fractured the tissue would remain in place. The white tissue allows subjective freedom of movement. The yellow elastic tissue can be stretched considerably while returning to its original length.

Tendons

Tendons are not elastic and are even less stretchy. Tendons are categorized as a connective tissue. Connective tissue supports, surrounds, and binds the muscle fibres. They contain both elastic and non-elastic tissue.

Areolar Tissue

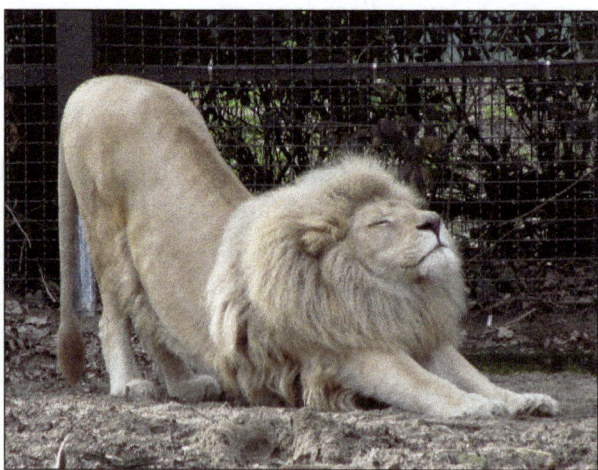
Stretching lion.

The areolar tissue is permeable and is extensively distributed throughout the body. This tissue acts as a general binder for all other tissues.

Muscle Tissue

Muscle tissue is made of a stretchy material. It is arranged in bundles of parallel fibres.

Stretch Receptors

Stretch receptors have two parts: Spindle cells and Golgi tendons. Spindle cells, located in the center of a muscle, send messages for the muscle to contract. On the other hand, Golgi tendon receptors are located near the end of a muscle fiber and send messages for the muscle to relax. As these receptors are trained through continual use, stretching becomes easier. When reflexes that inhibit flexibility are released the splits then become easier to perform. The splits use the body's complete range of motion and provide a complete stretch.

Limits of Flexibility

Each individual is born with a particular range of motion for each joint in their body. In the book Finding Balance by Gigi Berardi, the author mentions three limiting factors: Occupational demands, movement demands and training oversights.

Internal Factors of Flexibility

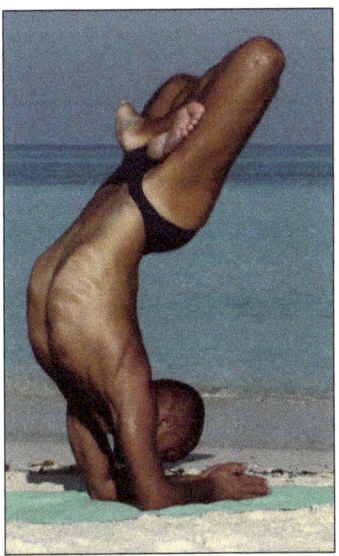

Male yoga practitioner in an inverted lotus position.

Movement demands include strength, endurance and range of motion. Training oversights occurs when the body is overused. Internally, the joints, muscles, tendons, and ligaments can affect one's flexibility. As previously mentioned, each part of the body has its own limitations and combined, the range of motion can be affected. The mental attitude of the performer during the state of motion can also affect their range.

External Factors of Flexibility

Externally, anything from the weather outside to the age of the performer can affect flexibility. General tissues and collagen change with age influencing the individual. As one ages, performing activities of daily living without pain becomes much harder. By stretching often, one can maintain a level of musculoskeletal fitness that will keep them feeling well.

Performers should be aware of over-stretching. Even basic things such as clothing and equipment can affect a performance. Dance surfaces and lack of proper shoes can also affect a performer's ability to perform at his/her best.

Signs of Injury

Stretching for too long or too much can give way to an injury. For most activities, the normal range of motion is more than adequate. Any sudden movements or going too fast can cause a muscle to tighten. This leads to extreme pain and the performer should let the muscle relax by resting.

Risk of Injury

Some people get injuries while doing yoga and aerobics so one needs to be careful while doing it. While most stretching does not cause injury, it is said that quick, ballistic stretching can if it is done incorrectly. If a bone, muscle or any other part is stretched more than its capacity it may lead to dislocation, muscle pulls, etc. or something even more severe too.

Neurobiological Effects of Physical Exercise

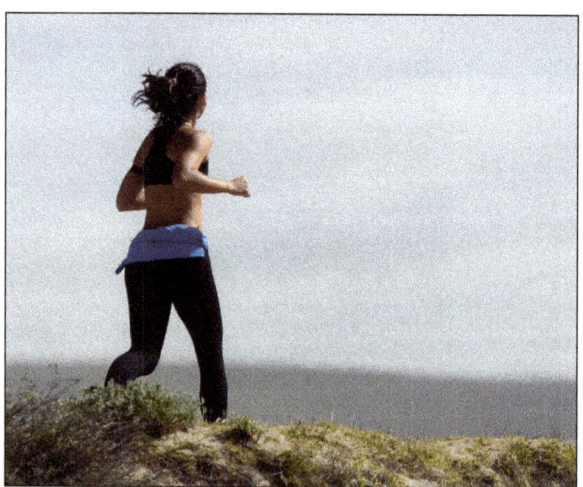
A woman engaging in aerobic exercise.

The neurobiological effects of physical exercise are numerous and involve a wide range of interrelated effects on brain structure, brain function, and cognition. A large body of research in humans has demonstrated that consistent aerobic exercise (e.g., 30 minutes every day) induces persistent improvements in certain cognitive functions, healthy alterations in gene expression in the brain, and beneficial forms of neuroplasticity and behavioral plasticity; some of these long-term effects include: increased neuron growth, increased neurological activity (e.g., c-Fos and BDNF signaling), improved stress coping, enhanced cognitive control of behavior, improved declarative, spatial, and working memory, and structural and functional improvements in brain structures and pathways associated with cognitive control and memory. The effects of exercise on cognition have important implications for improving academic performance in children and college students, improving adult productivity, preserving cognitive function in old age, preventing or treating certain neurological disorders, and improving overall quality of life.

In healthy adults, aerobic exercise has been shown to induce transient effects on cognition after a single exercise session and persistent effects on cognition following regular exercise over the course of several months. People who regularly perform aerobic exercise (e.g., running, jogging, brisk walking, swimming, and cycling) have greater scores on neuropsychological function and performance tests that measure certain cognitive functions, such as attentional control, inhibitory control, cognitive flexibility, working memory updating and capacity, declarative memory, spatial memory, and information processing speed. The transient effects of exercise on cognition include improvements in most executive functions (e.g., attention, working memory, cognitive flexibility, inhibitory control, problem solving, and decision making) and information processing speed for a period of up to 2 hours after exercising.

Aerobic exercise induces short- and long-term effects on mood and emotional states by promoting positive affect, inhibiting negative affect, and decreasing the biological response to acute psychological stress. Over the short-term, aerobic exercise functions as both an antidepressant and euphoriant, whereas consistent exercise produces general improvements in mood and self-esteem.

Regular aerobic exercise improves symptoms associated with a variety of central nervous system disorders and may be used as an adjunct therapy for these disorders. There is clear evidence of exercise treatment efficacy for major depressive disorder and attention deficit hyperactivity disorder. The American Academy of Neurology's clinical practice guideline for mild cognitive impairment indicates that clinicians should recommend regular exercise (two times per week) to individuals who have been diagnosed with this condition. Reviews of clinical evidence also support the use of exercise as an adjunct therapy for certain neurodegenerative disorders, particularly Alzheimer's disease and Parkinson's disease. Regular exercise is also associated with a lower risk of developing neurodegenerative disorders. A large body of preclinical evidence and emerging clinical evidence supports the use of exercise as an adjunct therapy for the treatment and prevention of drug addictions. Regular exercise has also been proposed as an adjunct therapy for brain cancers.

Long-term Effects

Neuroplasticity

Neuroplasticity is the process by which neurons adapt to a disturbance over time, and most often occurs in response to repeated exposure to stimuli. Aerobic exercise increases the production of neurotrophic factors (e.g., BDNF, IGF-1, VEGF) which mediate improvements in cognitive functions and various forms of memory by promoting blood vessel formation in the brain, adult neurogenesis, and other forms of neuroplasticity. Consistent aerobic exercise over a period of several months induces clinically significant improvements in executive functions and increased gray matter volume in nearly all regions of the brain, with the most marked increases occurring in brain regions that give rise to executive functions. The brain structures that show the greatest improvements in gray matter volume in response to aerobic exercise are the prefrontal cortex, caudate nucleus, and hippocampus; less significant increases in gray matter volume occur in the anterior cingulate cortex, parietal cortex, cerebellum, and nucleus accumbens. The prefrontal cortex, caudate nucleus, and anterior cingulate cortex are among the most significant brain structures in the dopamine and norepinephrine systems that give rise to cognitive control. Exercise-induced neurogenesis (i.e., the increases in gray matter volume) in the hippocampus is associated with measurable improvements in spatial memory. Higher physical fitness scores, as measured by VO_2 max, are associated with better executive function, faster information processing speed, and greater gray matter volume of the hippocampus, caudate nucleus, and nucleus accumbens. Long-term aerobic exercise is also associated with persistent beneficial epigenetic changes that result in improved stress coping, improved cognitive function, and increased neuronal activity (c-Fos and BDNF signaling).

Structural Growth

Neuroimaging studies indicate that consistent aerobic exercise increases gray matter volume in nearly all regions of the brain, with more pronounced increases occurring in brain regions associated with memory processing, cognitive control, motor function, and reward; the most prominent gains in gray matter volume are seen in the prefrontal cortex, caudate nucleus, and hippocampus, which support cognitive control and memory processing, among other cognitive functions. Moreover, the left and right halves of the prefrontal cortex, the hippocampus, and the cingulate cortex appear to become more functionally interconnected in response to consistent aerobic exercise. Three reviews indicate that marked improvements in prefrontal and hippocampal gray matter volume occur in healthy adults that regularly engage in medium intensity exercise for several months. Other regions of the brain that demonstrate moderate or less significant gains in gray matter volume during neuroimaging include the anterior cingulate cortex, parietal cortex, cerebellum, and nucleus accumbens.

Regular exercise has been shown to counter the shrinking of the hippocampus and memory impairment that naturally occurs in late adulthood. Sedentary adults over age 55 show a 1–2% decline in hippocampal volume annually. A neuroimaging study with a sample of 120 adults revealed that participating in regular aerobic exercise increased the volume of the left hippocampus by 2.12% and the right hippocampus by 1.97% over a one-year period. Subjects in the low intensity stretching group who had higher fitness levels at baseline showed less hippocampal volume loss, providing evidence for exercise being protective against age-related cognitive decline. In general, individuals that exercise more over a given period have greater hippocampal volumes and better memory function. Aerobic exercise has also been shown to induce growth in the white matter tracts in the anterior corpus callosum, which normally shrink with age.

The various functions of the brain structures that show exercise-induced increases in gray matter volume include:

- Prefrontal and anterior cingulate cortices: Required for the cognitive control of behavior, particularly, working memory, attentional control, decision-making, cognitive flexibility, social cognition, and inhibitory control of behavior; implicated in attention deficit hyperactivity disorder (ADHD) and addiction.

- Nucleus accumbens: Responsible for incentive salience ("wanting" or desire, the form of motivation associated with reward) and positive reinforcement; implicated in addiction.

- Hippocampus: Responsible for storage and consolidation of declarative memory and spatial memory; implicated in depression.

- Cerebellum: Responsible for motor coordination and motor learning.

- Caudate nucleus: Responsible for stimulus-response learning and inhibitory control; implicated in Parkinson's disease and ADHD.

- Parietal cortex: Responsible for sensory perception, working memory, and attention.

Persistent Effects on Cognition

Concordant with the functional roles of the brain structures that exhibit increased gray matter volumes, regular exercise over a period of several months has been shown to persistently improve numerous executive functions and several forms of memory. In particular, consistent aerobic exercise has been shown to improve attentional control, information processing speed, cognitive flexibility (e.g., task switching), inhibitory control, working memory updating and capacity, declarative memory, and spatial memory. In healthy young and middle-aged adults, the effect sizes of improvements in cognitive function are largest for indices of executive functions and small to moderate for aspects of memory and information processing speed. It may be that in older adults, individuals benefit cognitively by taking part in both aerobic and resistance type exercise of at least moderate intensity. Individuals who have a sedentary lifestyle tend to have impaired executive functions relative to other more physically active non-exercisers. A reciprocal relationship between exercise and executive functions has also been noted: improvements in executive control processes, such as attentional control and inhibitory control, increase an individual's tendency to exercise.

Mechanism of Effects

BDNF Signaling

One of the most significant effects of exercise on the brain is the increased synthesis and expression of BDNF, a neuropeptide and hormone, in the brain and periphery, resulting in increased signaling through its receptor tyrosine kinase, tropomyosin receptor kinase B (TrkB). Since, BDNF is capable of crossing the blood–brain barrier, higher peripheral BDNF synthesis also increases BDNF signaling in the brain. Exercise-induced increases in brain BDNF signaling are associated with beneficial epigenetic changes, improved cognitive function, improved mood, and improved memory. Furthermore, research has provided a great deal of support for the role of BDNF in hippocampal neurogenesis, synaptic plasticity, and neural repair. Engaging in moderate-high intensity aerobic exercise such as running, swimming, and cycling increases BDNF biosynthesis through myokine signaling, resulting in up to a threefold increase in blood plasma and brain BDNF levels; exercise intensity is positively correlated with the magnitude of increased BDNF biosynthesis and expression. A meta-analysis of studies involving the effect of exercise on BDNF levels found that consistent exercise modestly increases resting BDNF levels as well. This has important implications for exercise as a mechanism to reduce stress since stress is closely linked with decreased levels of BDNF in the hippocampus. In fact, studies suggest that BDNF contributes to the anxiety-reducing effects of antidepressants. The increase in BDNF levels caused by exercise helps reverse the stress-induced decrease in BDNF which mediates stress in the short term and buffers against stress-related diseases in the long term.

IGF-1 Signaling

IGF-1 is a peptide and neurotrophic factor that mediates some of the effects of growth hormone; IGF-1 elicits its physiological effects by binding to a specific receptor tyrosine kinase, the IGF-1 receptor, to control tissue growth and remodeling. In the brain, IGF-1 functions as a neurotrophic factor that, like BDNF, plays a significant role in cognition, neurogenesis, and neuronal survival. Physical activity is associated with increased levels of IGF-1 in blood serum, which is known to contribute to neuroplasticity in the brain due to its capacity to cross the blood–brain barrier and blood–cerebrospinal fluid barrier; consequently, one review noted that IGF-1 is a key mediator of exercise-induced adult neurogenesis, while a second review characterized it as a factor which links "body fitness" with "brain fitness". The amount of IGF-1 released into blood plasma during exercise is positively correlated with exercise intensity and duration.

VEGF Signaling

VEGF is a neurotrophic and angiogenic (i.e., blood vessel growth-promoting) signaling protein that binds to two receptor tyrosine kinases, VEGFR1 and VEGFR2, which are expressed in neurons and glial cells in the brain. Hypoxia, or inadequate cellular oxygen supply, strongly upregulates VEGF expression and VEGF exerts a neuroprotective effect in hypoxic neurons. Like BDNF and IGF-1, aerobic exercise has been shown to increase VEGF biosynthesis in peripheral tissue which subsequently crosses the blood–brain barrier and promotes neurogenesis and blood vessel formation in the central nervous system. Exercise-induced increases in VEGF signaling have been shown to improve cerebral blood volume and contribute to exercise-induced neurogenesis in the hippocampus.

Short-term Effects

Transient Effects on Cognition

In addition to the persistent effects on cognition that result from several months of daily exercise, acute exercise (i.e., a single bout of exercise) has been shown to transiently improve a number of cognitive functions. Reviews and meta-analyses of research on the effects of acute exercise on cognition in healthy young and middle-aged adults have concluded that information processing speed and a number of executive functions – including attention, working memory, problem solving, cognitive flexibility, verbal fluency, decision making, and inhibitory control – all improve for a period of up to 2 hours post-exercise. A systematic review of studies conducted on children also suggested that some of the exercise-induced improvements in executive function are apparent after single bouts of exercise, while other aspects (e.g., attentional control) only improve following consistent exercise on a regular basis. Other research has suggested performative enhancements during exercise, such as exercise-concurrent improvements in processing speed during visual working memory tasks.

Exercise-induced Euphoria

Continuous exercise can produce a transient state of euphoria – a positively-valenced affective state involving the experience of pleasure and feelings of profound contentment, elation, and well-being – which is colloquially known as a "runner's high" in distance running or a "rower's high" in rowing. Current medical reviews indicate that several endogenous euphoriants are responsible for producing exercise-related euphoria, specifically phenethylamine (an endogenous psychostimulant), β-endorphin (an endogenous opioid), and anandamide (an endogenous cannabinoid).

Effects on Neurochemistry

β-Phenylethylamine

β-Phenylethylamine, commonly referred to as *phenethylamine,* is a human trace amine and potent catecholaminergic and glutamatergic neuromodulator that has similar psychostimulant and euphoriant effects and a similar chemical structure to amphetamine. Thirty minutes of moderate to high intensity physical exercise has been shown to induce an enormous increase in urinary β-phenylacetic acid, the primary metabolite of phenethylamine. The average 24 hour urinary β-phenylacetic acid concentration among participants following just 30 minutes of intense exercise increased by 77% relative to baseline concentrations in resting control subjects; the reviews suggest that phenethylamine synthesis sharply increases while an individual is exercising, during which time it is rapidly metabolized due to its short half-life of roughly 30 seconds. In a resting state, phenethylamine is synthesized in catecholamine neurons from L-phenylalanine by aromatic amino acid decarboxylase (AADC) at approximately the same rate at which dopamine is produced.

In humans, catecholamines and phenethylaminergic trace amines are derived from the amino acid L-phenylalanine.

In light of this observation, the original paper and both reviews suggest that phenethylamine plays a prominent role in mediating the mood-enhancing euphoric effects of a runner's high, as both phenethylamine and amphetamine are potent euphoriants.

β-Endorphin

β-Endorphin (contracted from "endogenous morphine") is an endogenous opioid neuropeptide that binds to μ-opioid receptors, in turn producing euphoria and pain relief. A meta-analytic review found that exercise significantly increases the secretion of β-endorphin and that this secretion is correlated with improved mood states. Moderate intensity exercise produces the greatest increase in β-endorphin synthesis, while higher and lower intensity forms of exercise are associated with smaller increases in β-endorphin synthesis. A review on β-endorphin and exercise noted that an individual's mood improves for the remainder of the day following physical exercise and that one's mood is positively correlated with overall daily physical activity level.

Anandamide

Anandamide is an endogenous cannabinoid and retrograde neurotransmitter that binds to cannabinoid receptors (primarily CB_1), in turn producing euphoria. It has been shown that aerobic exercise causes an increase in plasma anandamide levels, where the magnitude of this increase is highest at moderate exercise intensity (i.e., exercising at ~70–80% maximum heart rate). Increases in plasma anandamide levels are associated with psychoactive effects because anandamide is able to cross the blood–brain barrier and act within the central nervous system. Thus, because anandamide is a euphoriant and aerobic exercise is associated with euphoric effects, it has been proposed that anandamide partly mediates the short-term mood-lifting effects of exercise (e.g., the euphoria of a runner's high) via exercise-induced increases in its synthesis.

In mice, it was demonstrated that certain features of a runner's high depend on cannabinoid receptors. Pharmacological or genetic disruption of cannabinoid signaling via cannabinoid receptors prevents the analgesic and anxiety-reducing effects of running.

Cortisol and the Psychological Stress Response

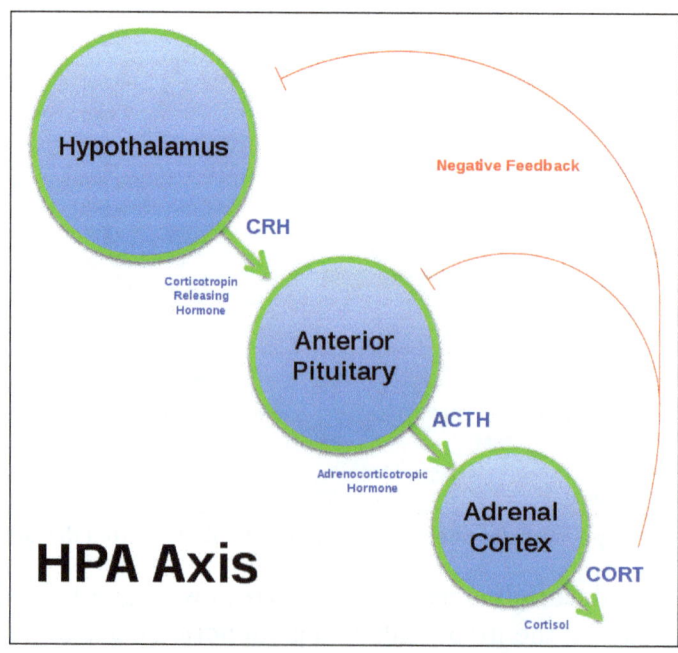

Diagram of the hypothalamic–pituitary–adrenal axis.

The "stress hormone", cortisol, is a glucocorticoid that binds to glucocorticoid receptors. Psychological stress induces the release of cortisol from the adrenal gland by activating the hypothalamic–pituitary–adrenal axis (HPA axis). Short-term increases in cortisol levels are associated with adaptive cognitive improvements, such as enhanced inhibitory control; however, excessively high exposure or prolonged exposure to high levels of cortisol causes impairments in cognitive control and has neurotoxic effects in the human brain. For example, chronic psychological stress decreases BDNF expression which has detrimental effects on hippocampal volume and can lead to depression.

As a physical stressor, aerobic exercise stimulates cortisol secretion in an intensity-dependent manner; however, it does not result in long-term increases in cortisol production since this exercise-induced effect on cortisol is a response to transient negative energy balance. Individuals who have recently exercised exhibit improvements in stress coping behaviors. Aerobic exercise increases physical fitness and lowers neuroendocrine (i.e., HPA axis) reactivity and therefore reduces the biological response to psychological stress in humans (e.g., reduced cortisol release and attenuated heart rate response). Exercise also reverses stress-induced decreases in BDNF expression and signaling in the brain, thereby acting as a buffer against stress-related diseases like depression.

Glutamate and GABA

Glutamate, one of the most common neurochemicals in the brain, is an excitatory neurotransmitter involved in many aspects of brain function, including learning and memory. Based upon animal models, exercise appears to normalize the excessive levels of glutamate neurotransmission into the nucleus accumbens that occurs in drug addiction. A review of the effects of exercise on neurocardiac function in preclinical models noted that exercise-induced neuroplasticity of the rostral ventrolateral medulla (RVLM) has an inhibitory effect on glutamatergic neurotransmission in this region, in turn reducing sympathetic activity; the review hypothesized that this neuroplasticity in the RVLM is a mechanism by which regular exercise prevents inactivity-related cardiovascular disease.

Effects on Central Nervous System Disorders

Addiction

Clinical and preclinical evidence indicate that consistent aerobic exercise, especially endurance exercise (e.g., marathon running), actually prevents the development of certain drug addictions and is an effective adjunct treatment for drug addiction, and psychostimulant addiction in particular. Consistent aerobic exercise magnitude-dependently (i.e., by duration and intensity) reduces drug addiction risk, which appears to occur through the reversal of drug-induced, addiction-related neuroplasticity. Exercise may prevent the development of drug addiction by altering ΔFosB or c-Fos immunoreactivity in the striatum or other parts of the reward system. Moreover, aerobic exercise decreases psychostimulant self-administration, reduces the reinstatement (i.e., relapse) of drug-seeking, and induces opposite effects on striatal dopamine receptor D_2 (DRD2) signaling (increased DRD2 density) to those induced by pathological stimulant use (decreased DRD2 density). Consequently, consistent aerobic exercise may lead to better treatment outcomes when used as an adjunct treatment for drug addiction. As of 2016, more clinical research is still needed to understand the mechanisms and confirm the efficacy of exercise in drug addiction treatment and prevention.

Attention Deficit Hyperactivity Disorder

Regular physical exercise, particularly aerobic exercise, is an effective add-on treatment for ADHD in children and adults, particularly when combined with stimulant medication (i.e., amphetamine or methylphenidate), although the best intensity and type of aerobic exercise for improving symptoms are not currently known. In particular, the long-term effects of regular aerobic exercise in ADHD individuals include better behavior and motor abilities, improved executive functions (including attention, inhibitory control, and planning, among other cognitive domains), faster information processing speed, and better memory. Parent-teacher ratings of behavioral and socio-emotional outcomes in response to regular aerobic exercise include: better overall function, reduced ADHD symptoms, better self-esteem, reduced levels of anxiety and depression, fewer somatic complaints, better academic and classroom behavior, and improved social behavior. Exercising while on stimulant medication augments the effect of stimulant medication on executive function. It is believed that these short-term effects of exercise are mediated by an increased abundance of synaptic dopamine and norepinephrine in the brain.

Major Depressive Disorder

A number of medical reviews have indicated that exercise has a marked and persistent antidepressant effect in humans, an effect believed to be mediated through enhanced BDNF signaling in the brain. Several systematic reviews have analyzed the potential for physical exercise in the treatment of depressive disorders. The 2013 Cochrane Collaboration review on physical exercise for depression noted that, based upon limited evidence, it is more effective than a control intervention and comparable to psychological or antidepressant drug therapies. Three subsequent 2014 systematic reviews that included the Cochrane review in their analysis concluded with similar findings: one indicated that physical exercise is effective as an adjunct treatment (i.e., treatments that are used together) with antidepressant medication; the other two indicated that physical exercise has marked antidepressant effects and recommended the inclusion of physical activity as an adjunct treatment for mild–moderate depression and mental illness in general. One systematic review noted that yoga may be effective in alleviating symptoms of prenatal depression.

A 2015 clinical evidence which included a medical guideline for the treatment of depression with exercise noted that the available evidence on the effectiveness of exercise therapy for depression suffers from some limitations; nonetheless, it stated that there is clear evidence of efficacy for reducing symptoms of depression. The review also noted that patient characteristics, the type of depressive disorder, and the nature of the exercise program all affect the antidepressant properties of exercise therapy. A meta-analysis from July 2016 concluded that physical exercise improves overall quality of life in individuals with depression relative to controls.

Mild Cognitive Impairment

The American Academy of Neurology's January 2018 update of their clinical practice guideline for mild cognitive impairment states that clinicians should recommend regular exercise (two times per week) to individuals who have been diagnosed with this condition. This guidance is based upon a moderate amount of high-quality evidence which supports the efficacy of regular physical exercise (twice weekly over a 6-month period) for improving cognitive symptoms in individuals with mild cognitive impairment.

Neurodegenerative Disorders

Alzheimer's Disease

Alzheimer's Disease is a cortical neurodegenerative disorder and the most prevalent form of dementia, representing approximately 65% of all cases of dementia; it is characterized by impaired cognitive function, behavioral abnormalities, and a reduced capacity to perform basic activities of daily life. Two meta-analytic systematic reviews of randomized controlled trials with durations of 3–12 months have examined the effects of physical exercise on the aforementioned characteristics of Alzheimer's disease. The reviews found beneficial effects of physical exercise on cognitive function, the rate of cognitive decline, and the ability to perform activities of daily living in individuals with Alzheimer's disease. One review suggested that, based upon transgenic mouse models, the cognitive effects of exercise on Alzheimer's disease may result from a reduction in the quantity of amyloid plaque.

The Caerphilly Prospective study followed 2,375 male subjects over 30 years and examined the association between healthy lifestyles and dementia, among other factors. Analyses of the Caerphilly study data have found that exercise is associated with a lower incidence of dementia and a reduction in cognitive impairment. A subsequent systematic review of longitudinal studies also found higher levels of physical activity to be associated with a reduction in the risk of dementia and cognitive decline; this review further asserted that increased physical activity appears to be causally related with these reduced risks.

Parkinson's Disease

Parkinson's disease (PD) is a movement disorder that produces symptoms such as bradykinesia, rigidity, shaking, and impaired gait.

A review by Kramer and colleagues found that some neurotransmitter systems are affected by exercise in a positive way. A few studies reported seeing an improvement in brain health and cognitive function due to exercise. One particular study by Kramer and colleagues found that aerobic training improved executive control processes supported by frontal and prefrontal regions of the brain. These regions are responsible for the cognitive deficits in PD patients, however there was speculation that the difference in the neurochemical environment in the frontal lobes of PD patients may inhibit the benefit of aerobic exercise. Nocera and colleagues performed a case study based on this literature where they gave participants with early-to mid-staged PD, and the control group cognitive/language assessments with exercise regimens. Individuals performed 20 minutes of aerobic exercise three times a week for 8 weeks on a stationary exercise cycle. It was found that aerobic exercise improved several measures of cognitive function, providing evidence that such exercise regimens may be beneficial to patients with PD.

Delayed Onset Muscle Soreness

Delayed onset muscle soreness (DOMS) is the pain and stiffness felt in muscles several hours to days after unaccustomed or strenuous exercise.

The soreness is felt most strongly 24 to 72 hours after the exercise. It is thought to be caused by eccentric (lengthening) exercise, which causes small-scale damage (microtrauma) to the muscle fibers. After such exercise, the muscle adapts rapidly to prevent muscle damage, and thereby soreness, if the exercise is repeated.

Delayed onset muscle soreness is one symptom of exercise-induced muscle damage. The other is acute muscle soreness, which appears during and immediately after exercise.

Signs and Symptoms

The soreness is perceived as a dull, aching pain in the affected muscle, often combined with tenderness and stiffness. The pain is typically felt only when the muscle is stretched, contracted or put under pressure, not when it is at rest. This tenderness, a characteristic symptom of DOMS, is also referred to as "muscular mechanical hyperalgesia".

Although there is variance among exercises and individuals, the soreness usually increases in intensity in the first 24 hours after exercise. It peaks from 24 to 72 hours, then subsides and disappears up to seven days after exercise.

Cause

The muscle soreness is caused by eccentric exercise, that is, exercise consisting of eccentric (lengthening) contractions of the muscle. Isometric (static) exercise causes much less soreness, and concentric (shortening) exercise causes none.

Mechanism

The mechanism of delayed onset muscle soreness is not completely understood, but the pain is ultimately thought to be a result of microtrauma – mechanical damage at a very small scale – to the muscles being exercised.

DOMS was first described in 1902 by Theodore Hough, who concluded that this kind of soreness is "fundamentally the result of ruptures within the muscle". According to this "muscle damage" theory of DOMS, these ruptures are microscopic lesions at the Z-line of the muscle sarcomere. The soreness has been attributed to the increased tension force and muscle lengthening from eccentric exercise. This may cause the actin and myosin cross-bridges to separate prior to relaxation, ultimately causing greater tension on the remaining active motor units. This increases the risk of broadening, smearing, and damage to the sarcomere. When microtrauma occurs to these structures, nociceptors (pain receptors) within the muscle's connective tissues are stimulated and cause a sensation of pain.

Another explanation for the pain associated with DOMS is the "enzyme efflux" theory. Following microtrauma, calcium that is normally stored in the sarcoplasmic reticulum accumulates in the damaged muscles. Cellular respiration is inhibited and ATP needed to actively transport calcium back into the sarcoplasmic reticulum is also slowed. This accumulation of calcium may activate proteases and phospholipases which in turn break down and degenerate muscle protein. This causes inflammation, and in turn pain due to the accumulation of histamines, prostaglandins, and potassium.

An earlier theory posited that DOMS is connected to the build-up of lactic acid in the blood, which was thought to continue being produced following exercise. This build-up of lactic acid was thought to be a toxic metabolic waste product that caused the perception of pain at a delayed stage. This theory has been largely rejected, as concentric contractions which also produce lactic acid have been unable to cause DOMS. Additionally, lactic acid is known from multiple studies to return to normal levels within one hour of exercise, and therefore cannot cause the pain that occurs much later.

Relation to other Effects

Although delayed onset muscle soreness is a symptom associated with muscle damage, its magnitude does not necessarily reflect the magnitude of muscle damage.

Soreness is one of the temporary changes caused in muscles by unaccustomed eccentric exercise. Other such changes include decreased muscle strength, reduced range of motion, and muscle swelling. It has been shown, however, that these changes develop independently in time from one another and that the soreness is therefore not the cause of the reduction in muscle function.

Possible Function as a Warning Sign

Soreness might conceivably serve as a warning to reduce muscle activity to prevent injury or further injury. With delayed onset muscle soreness (DOMS) caused by eccentric exercise (muscle lengthening), it was observed that light concentric exercise (muscle shortening) during DOMS can cause initially more pain but was followed by a temporary alleviation of soreness – with no adverse effects on muscle function or recovery being observed. Furthermore eccentric exercise during DOMS was found to not exacerbate muscle damage, nor did it have an adverse effect on recovery – considering this, soreness is not necessarily a warning sign to reduce the usage of the affected muscle. However it was observed that a second bout of eccentric exercise within one week of the initial exercise did lead to decreased muscle function immediately afterwards.

Repeated-bout Effect

After performing an unaccustomed eccentric exercise and exhibiting severe soreness, the muscle rapidly adapts to reduce further damage from the same exercise. This is called the "repeated-bout effect".

As a result of this effect, not only is the soreness reduced, but other indicators of muscle damage, such as swelling, reduced strength and reduced range of motion, are also more quickly recovered from. The effect is mostly, but not wholly, specific to the exercised muscle: experiments have shown that some of the protective effect is also conferred on other muscles.

The magnitude of the effect is subject to many variations, depending for instance on the time between bouts, the number and length of eccentric contractions and the exercise mode. It also varies between people and between indicators of muscle damage. Generally, though, the protective effect lasts for at least several weeks. It seems to gradually decrease as time between bouts increases, and is undetectable after about one year.

The first bout does not need to be as intense as the subsequent bouts in order to confer at least some protection against soreness. For instance, eccentric exercise performed at 40% of maximal strength has been shown to confer a protection of 20 to 60% from muscle damage incurred by a 100% strength exercise two to three weeks later. Also, the repeated-bout effect appears even after a relatively small number of contractions, possibly as few as two. In one study, a first bout of 10, 20 or 50 contractions provided equal protection for a second bout of 50 contractions three weeks later.

The reason for the protective effect is not yet understood. A number of possible mechanisms, which may complement one another, have been proposed. These include neural adaptations (improved use and control of the muscle by the nervous system), mechanical adaptations (increased muscle stiffness or muscle support tissue), and cellular adaptations (adaptation to inflammatory response and increased protein synthesis, among others).

Prevention

Delayed onset muscle soreness can be reduced or prevented by gradually increasing the intensity of a new exercise program, thereby taking advantage of the repeated-bout effect. Soreness can theoretically be avoided by limiting exercise to concentric and isometric contractions. But eccentric contractions in some muscles are normally unavoidable during exercise, especially when muscles are fatigued. Limiting the length of eccentric muscle extensions during exercise may afford some protection against soreness, but this may also not be practical depending on the mode of exercise. Static stretching or warming up the muscles before or after exercise does not prevent soreness.

Treatment

The soreness usually disappears within about 72 hours after appearing. If treatment is desired, any measure that increases blood flow to the muscle, such as low-intensity activity, massage, nerve mobilization, hot baths, or a sauna visit may help somewhat.

Immersion in cool or icy water, an occasionally recommended remedy, was found to be ineffective in alleviating DOMS in one 2011 study, but effective in another. There is also insufficient evidence to determine whether whole-body cryotherapy – compared with passive rest or no whole-body cryotherapy – reduces DOMS, or improves subjective recovery, after exercise.

Counterintuitively, continued exercise may temporarily suppress the soreness. Exercise increases pain thresholds and pain tolerance. This effect, called exercise-induced analgesia, is known to occur in endurance training (running, cycling, swimming), but little is known about whether it also occurs in resistance training. There are claims in the literature that exercising sore muscles appears to be the best way to reduce or eliminate the soreness, but this has not yet been systematically investigated.

Exercise-induced Bronchoconstriction

Exercise-induced asthma, or E.I.A., occurs when the airways narrow as a result of exercise. The preferred term for this condition is exercise-induced bronchoconstriction (EIB); exercise does not cause asthma, but is frequently an asthma trigger.

Signs and Symptoms

It might be expected that people with E.I.B. would present with shortness of breath, and/or an elevated respiratory rate and wheezing, consistent with an asthma attack. However, many will present with decreased stamina, or difficulty in recovering from exertion compared to team members, or paroxysmal coughing from an irritable airway. Similarly, examination may reveal wheezing and prolonged expiratory phase, or may be quite normal. Consequently, a potential for under-diagnosis exists. Measurement of airflow, such as peak expiratory flow rates, which can be done inexpensively on the track or sideline, may prove helpful.

Cause

While the potential triggering events for E.I.B. are well recognized, the underlying pathogenesis is poorly understood. It usually occurs after at least several minutes of vigorous, aerobic activity, which increases oxygen demand to the point where breathing through the nose (nasal breathing) must be supplemented by mouth breathing. The resultant inhalation of air that has not been warmed and humidified by the nasal passages seems to generate increased blood flow to the linings of the bronchial tree, resulting in edema. Constriction of these small airways then follows, worsening the degree of obstruction to airflow. There is increasing evidence that the smooth muscle that lines the airways becomes progressively more sensitive to changes that occur as a result of injury to the airways from dehydration. The chemical mediators that provoke the muscle spasm appear to arise from mast cells.

Diagnosis

Exercise-induced bronchoconstriction can be difficult to diagnose clinically given the lack of specific symptoms and frequent misinterpretation as manifestations of vigorous exercise. There are many mimics that present with similar symptoms, such as vocal cord dysfunction, cardiac arrhythmias, cardiomyopathies, and gastroesophageal reflux disease. It is also important to distinguish those who have asthma with exercise worsening, and who consequently will have abnormal testing at rest, from true exercise-induced bronchoconstriction, where there will be normal baseline results. Because of the wide differential diagnosis of exertional respiratory complaints, the diagnosis of exercise-induced bronchoconstriction based on history and self-reported symptoms alone has been shown to be inaccurate and will result in an incorrect diagnosis more than 50% of the time. An important and often over-looked differential diagnosis is exercise-induced laryngeal obstruction EILO. The latter can co-exist with EIB and is best differentiated using objective testing and continuous laryngoscopy during exercise (CLE) testing.

Spirometry

Objective testing should begin with spirometry at rest. In true exercise-induced bronchoconstriction, the results should be within normal limits. Should resting values be abnormal, then asthma, or some other chronic lung condition, is present. There is, of course, no reason why asthma and exercise-induced bronchoconstriction should not co-exist but the distinction is important because without successful treatment of underlying asthma, treatment of an exercise component will likely be unsuccessful. If baseline testing is normal, some form of exercise or pharmacologic stress will be required, either on the sideline or practice venue, or in the laboratory.

Exercise Testing

Treadmill or ergometer-based testing in lung function laboratories are effective methods for diagnosing exercise-induced bronchoconstriction, but may result in false negatives if the exercise stimulus is not intense enough.

Field-exercise Challenge

Field-exercise challenge tests that involve the athlete performing the sport in which they are normally involved and assessing FEV_1 after exercise are helpful if abnormal but have been shown to be less sensitive than eucapnic voluntary hyperventilation.

Eucapnic Voluntary Hyperventilation Challenge

The International Olympic Committee recommends the eucapnic voluntary hyperventilation (EVH) challenge as the test to document exercise-induced asthma in Olympic athletes. In the EVH challenge, the patient voluntarily, without exercising, rapidly breathes dry air enriched with 5% CO_2 for six minutes. The presence of the enriched CO_2 compensates for the CO_2 losses in the expired air, not matched by metabolic production, that occurs during hyperventilation, and so maintains CO_2 levels at normal.

Medication Challenge

Medication challenge tests, such as the methacholine challenge test, have a lower sensitivity for detection of exercise-induced bronchoconstriction in athletes and are also not a recommended first-line approach in the evaluation of exercise-induced asthma.

Mannitol inhalation has been recently approved for use in the United States.

A relatively recent review of the literature has concluded that there is currently insufficient available evidence to conclude that either mannitol inhalation or eucapnic voluntary hyperventilation are suitable alternatives to exercise challenge testing to detect exercise-induced bronchoconstriction and that additional research is required.

Treatment

Lifestyle

The best treatment is avoidance of conditions predisposing to attacks, when possible. In athletes who wish to continue their sport or do so in adverse conditions, preventive measures include altered training techniques and medications.

Some take advantage of the refractory period by precipitating an attack by "warming up," and then timing competition such that it occurs during the refractory period. Step-wise training works in a similar fashion. Warm up occurs in stages of increasing intensity, using the refractory period generated by each stage to reach a full workload.

Medication

The treatment of EIB has been extensively studied in asthmatic subjects over the last 30 years, but not so in EIB. Thus, it is not known whether athletes with EIB or 'sports asthma' respond similarly to subjects with classical allergic or nonallergic asthma. However, there is no evidence supporting different treatment for EIB in asthmatic athletes and nonathletes.

The most common medication used is a beta agonist taken about 20 minutes before exercise. Some physicians prescribe inhaled anti-inflammatory mists such as corticosteroids or leukotriene antagonists, and mast cell stabilizers have also proven effective. A randomized crossover study compared oral montelukast with inhaled salmeterol, both given two hours before exercise. Both drugs had similar benefit but montelukast lasted 24 hours.

Three randomized double-blind cross-over trials have examined the effect of vitamin C on EIB. Pooling the results of the three vitamin C trials indicates an average 48% reduction in the FEV1 decline caused by exercise. The systematic review concluded that "given the safety and low cost of vitamin C, and the positive findings for vitamin C administration in the three EIB studies, it seems reasonable for physically active people to test vitamin C when they have respiratory symptoms such as cough associated with exercise." It should be acknowledged that the total number of subjects involved in all three trials was only 40.

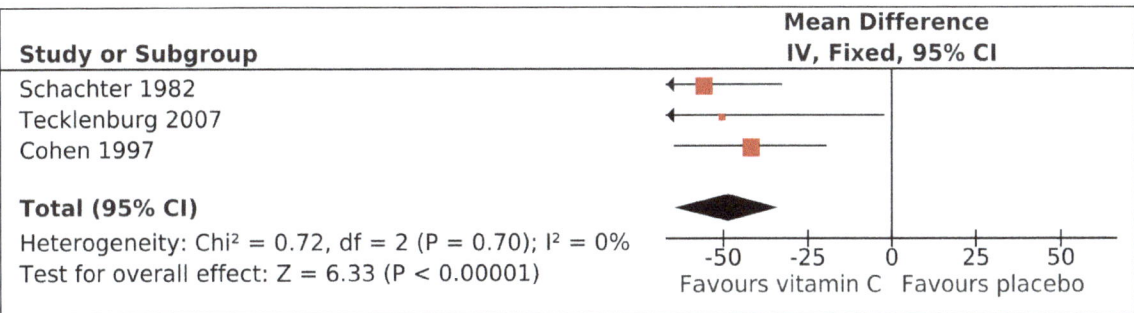

This forest plot shows the effect of vitamin C (0.5–2 g/day) on post-exercise decline in FEV1 in three studies with asthmatic participants. The three horizontal lines indicate the three studies, and the diamond shape at the bottom indicates the pooled effect of vitamin C: decrease in the post-exercise decline in FEV1 by 48% (95%CI: 33 to 64%).

In May 2013, the American Thoracic Society issued the first treatment guidelines for EIB.

Exercise-induced Laryngeal Obstruction

Exercise-induced laryngeal obstruction (EILO) is a transient, reversible narrowing of the larynx that occurs during high intensity exercise. This acts to impair airflow and cause shortness of breath, stridor and often discomfort in the throat and upper chest. EILO is a very common cause of breathing difficulties in young athletic individuals but is often misdiagnosed as asthma or exercise-induced bronchoconstriction.

Causes

EILO may arise because of a relative mechanical 'insufficiency' of the laryngeal structures that should act to maintain glottic patency.It has been proposed that a narrowing at the laryngeal inlet during the state of high airflow (e.g. when running fast), can act to cause a pressure drop across the larynx which then acts to 'pull' the laryngeal structures together. The Bernoulli principle states that increasing airflow through a tube creates increasing negative pressures within that tube.Complex neuromuscular functioning is required to maintain laryngeal opening and to allow the larynx to achieve a great number of tasks (i.e. speaking, airway protection, swallowing). It is, thus, also possible that EILO may arise as form a degree of neuromuscular failure. A small heredity study indicated that an autosomal dominant model of inheritance with variable expressivity and reduced penetrance in males may be relevant; because in ten families studied, there was at least one affected person in every generation in which both parents were examined. Further work is needed to determine if structural deficiencies in the laryngeal tissue of individuals with EILO are present.

Mechanism

EILO is typically caused by a narrowing of the supra-glottic structures of the larynx. In severe cases, these structures, also called arytenoids, can close over to almost completely close the laryngeal inlet. In fewer cases, the glottic (i.e. vocal cord) structures close together and this is typically what happens during exercise-induced vocal-cord dysfunction. EILO develops during intense exercise and closure develops as exercise becomes more intense. Closure of the voice box during exercise causes increased 'loading' on the breathing system and the respiratory muscles have to work much harder.

Epidemiology

The prevalence of EILO in adolescents and young adults appears to be in the range of 5–7% in northern Europe. Some, but not all studies report a higher female prevalence. Thus, in a study of 94 patients diagnosed using the CLE test, average age was ~15 years, and 68% were female. In athletic individuals EILO appears to be a highly prevalent cause of cough and wheeze and can co-exist with EIB. In one study, of almost 90 athletes, with unexplained respiratory symptoms, EILO was found to be present in approximately 30% of athletes, whilst EILO and EIB co-existed in one in ten. This condition can co-exist with other conditions, including severe asthma.

Clinical Features

- Key clinical features often include:
  - Difficulty 'catching a breath'.
  - Wheeze or whistling sound; typically when breathing in when exercising hard.
  - Throat or upper chest discomfort.
- Symptoms often start to improve from the time of exercise cessation / reducing exercise intensity.
- No improvement with standard asthma medication (e.g. salbutamol, albuterol).

Diagnosis

The current gold-standard means for diagnosing EILO is the continuous laryngoscopy during exercise test (CLE-test). This test involves the placement of a flexible laryngoscope via nostril, which is then secured in place and held with head-gear. It allows continuous visulization of the laryngeal aperture during exercise. The CLE test can be used during indoor treadmill or cycle-ergometer exercise but also whilst rowing or swimming or exercising outdoors There is a need to identify other less-invasive means of making a secure diagnosis. The examiner visually evaluates the relative change of the laryngeal inlet in the patien throughout the CLE-test. One common grading system uses 4 steps (0-3) on glottic and supraglottic level respectively. Grades (0-1) are considered normal, whereas grades (2-3) on either or both levels are consistent with EILO.

Exercise-associated Hyponatremia

Exercise-associated hyponatremia, is a fluid-electrolyte disorder caused by a decrease in sodium levels (hyponatremia) during or up to 24 hours after prolonged physical activity. This disorder can develop when marathon runners or endurance event athletes drink more fluid, usually water or sports drinks, than their kidneys can excrete. This excess water can severely dilute the level of sodium in the blood needed for organs, especially the brain, to function properly.

The incidence of EAH in athletes has increased in recent years, especially in the United States, as marathon races and endurance events have become more popular. A recent study showed 13% of the Boston 2002 marathon runners experienced EAH; most cases were mild. Eight deaths from EAH have been documented since 1985.

Symptoms

Symptoms may be absent or mild for the early onset of EAH and can include impaired exercise performance, nausea, vomiting, headache, bloating, and swelling of hands, legs, and feet. As water retention increases, weight gain may also occur. More severe symptoms include pulmonary edema and hyponatremic encephalopathy. Symptoms of hyponatremic encephalopathy are associated with an altered level of consciousness and can include sullenness, sleepiness, withdrawing from social interaction, photophobia, and seizures.

Causes

The primary causes of EAH include excessive fluid retention during exercise with a significant sodium deficit and excessive fluid intake leading to an increase in total body water resulting in a reduction in blood sodium levels.

Athlete-specific risk factors are: being of female sex; use of non-steroidal anti-inflammatory drugs [NSAIDs]; slow running; excessive fluid ingestion; low body weight; and event inexperience. Event-specific risk factors are: high availability of drinking fluids; duration of exercise exceeds 4 hours; unusually hot environmental conditions; and extreme cold temperature.

Mechanism

Sodium is an important electrolyte needed for maintaining blood pressure. Sodium is mainly found in the body fluids that surround the cells and is necessary for nerves, muscles, and other body tissues to function properly.

Many factors may contribute to the development of EAH. Under normal conditions, sodium and water levels are regulated by the renal and hormonal systems. The decrease in sodium levels can occur due to a defect in the renal and hormonal systems, an overwhelming increase in water consumption and excessive loss of sodium through sweating. When the sodium levels outside of the cells decrease, water moves into the cells. The cells begin to increase in size. When several cells in one area begin to increase in size, swelling occurs in the affected area. Swelling is commonly observed in hands, legs, and feet.

Sodium is also important in regulating the amount of water that passes through the blood-brain barrier. Decreased sodium blood levels result in increased permeability of water across the blood-brain barrier. This increased influx of water causes brain swelling which leads to severe neurological symptoms.

Diagnosis

EAH is categorized by having a blood serum or plasma sodium level below normal, which is less than 135 mmol/l. Asymptomatic EAH is not normally detected unless the athlete has had a sodium blood serum or plasma test. Hyponatremic encephalopathy may be detect using brain imaging studies and pulmonary edema may be confirmed by x-ray.

Prevention

Traditional prevention of EAH focuses on reducing fluid consumption to avoid fluid retention before, during, and after exercise.

However, since this can risk dehydration, an alternative approach is possible of consuming a substantial amount of salt prior to exercise. It is still important not to overconsume water to the extent of requiring urination, because urination would cause the extra salt to be excreted.

The Role of Thirst

In a published statement of the Third International Exercise-Associated Hyponatremia Consensus Development Conference, researchers concluded that drinking in accordance with the sensation of thirst is sufficient for preventing both dehydration and hyponatremia. This advice is contradicted by the American College of Sports Medicine, which has previously recommended athletes drink as much as tolerable. In October of 2015, ACSM President W. Larry Kenney stated that, "The clear and important health message should be that thirst alone is not the best indicator of dehydration or the body's fluid needs."

Brad L. Bennett, PhD claimed "perpetuation of the myth that one needs to drink beyond the dictates of thirst can be deadly." Similarly, authors of the Statement of the Third International Exercise-Associated Hyponatremia Consensus Development Conference claim this advice has "facilitated inadvertent overdrinking and pathological dilutional EAH."

Critics of the ACSM's view have questioned their motives, pointing out that Gatorade is one of the organizations "platinum sponsors."

Muscle Fatigue

At the start of exercising or when performing tasks, your muscles feel strong and resilient. However, over time and after repeating movements, your muscles may begin to feel weaker and tired. This can be defined as muscle fatigue.

Muscle fatigue is a symptom that decreases your muscles' ability to perform over time. It can be associated with a state of exhaustion, often following strenuous activity or exercise. When you experience fatigue, the force behind your muscles' movements decrease, causing you to feel weaker.

While exercise is a common cause of muscle fatigue, this symptom can be the result of other health conditions, too.

Causes of Muscle Fatigue

Exercise and other physical activity are a common cause of muscle fatigue. Other possible causes of this symptom include:

- Addison's disease
- Age
- Anaerobic infections
- Anemia
- Anxiety
- Botulism
- Cerebral palsy
- Chemotherapy
- Chronic fatigue syndrome (CFS)
- Dehydration
- Depression
- Fibromyalgia
- Hepatitis C
- HIV

- Hypothyroidism

- Influenza (the flu)

- Lack of exercise

- Lactic acid production

- Medications

- Mineral deficiency

- Muscular dystrophy

- Myasthenia gravis

- Myositis (muscle inflammation)

- Poor muscle tone due to a medical condition

- Pregnancy

- Sleep deprivation

- Stroke

- Tuberculosis

Muscle Fatigue Symptoms

Muscle fatigue can occur anywhere on the body. An initial sign of this condition is muscle weakness. Other symptoms associated with muscle fatigue include:

- Soreness

- Localized pain

- Shortness of breath

- Muscle twitching

- Trembling

- A weak grip

- Muscle cramps

If you begin having difficulty performing daily tasks or if your symptoms worsen, seek immediate medical attention. This could be an indication of a more serious health condition.

Outlook

Muscle fatigue decreases the amount of force you use to perform muscle actions. This symptom is often considered no cause for alarm unless your fatigue doesn't improve with rest.

In more severe cases, muscle fatigue can be an indication of a more serious disorder. Left untreated, this condition can lead to overwork and increase your risk of injury. Do not self-diagnose. If your muscle fatigue is paired with other irregular symptoms or if your condition doesn't improve after a few days, schedule a visit with your doctor.

Exercise-associated Muscle Cramps

Exercise-associated muscle cramps (EAMC) are a common condition experienced by recreational and competitive athletes. Despite their commonality and prevalence, their cause remains unknown. Theories for the cause of EAMC are primarily based on anecdotal and observational studies rather than sound experimental evidence. Without a clear cause, treatments and prevention strategies for EAMC are often unsuccessful.

Skeletal muscle cramps that occur during or shortly following exercise in healthy individuals with no underlying metabolic, neurological, or endocrine pathology have been termed exercise-associated muscle cramps (EAMC). Though controversial, an important differentiation in determining the cause of EAMC may be the number and location of muscles affected. EAMC typically occur in single, multijoint muscles (eg, triceps surae, quadriceps, hamstrings) when contracting in a shortened state, whereas generalized EAMC occur in multiple, usually bilateral muscles. Clinically, EAMC may be recognized by acute pain, stiffness, visible bulging or knotting of the muscle, and possible soreness that can last for several days. Although EAMC can be isolated, athletes often complain of EAMC symptoms up to 8 hours after exercise. This postexercise period of increased susceptibility to EAMC has been termed the cramp prone state. Although some EAMC do not appear to affect athletic performance, other times, EAMC can be completely debilitating.

A better understanding of the underlying mechanisms causing EAMC may allow better prevention and treatments, thus reducing the incidence rate. Norris et al. reported that 95% of physical education students (115 of 121) had experienced spontaneous cramps in their lifetimes with 26% (31 of 121) experiencing cramps after exercise. Kantarowski et al reported that 67% of triathletes (1631 of 2438) complained of EAMC under a variety of training conditions. More recently, a subset of American football players who experienced exertional heat illness reported concomitant skeletal muscle cramping. Thus, EAMC are common in both the recreational and the competitive athlete.

Although EAMC are common in athletes, the cause is unknown and controversial. Traditionally thought to be caused by factors associated with exercise in hot and humid environments (eg, dehydration and/or electrolyte imbalances), evidence suggests a neuromuscular cause. The inference from several studies is that EAMC have a singular, unknown cause. Authors have also suggested that there may be different kinds of EAMC and thus different causes (eg, isolated and generalized). Without a clear cause, the treatments and prevention strategies for EAMC vary considerably and have limited perceived effectiveness by health professionals. One approach to determining cause and the effectiveness of treatments is to examine the published studies and determine their level of evidence.

Theories for the Cause of EAMC

The dehydration–electrolyte imbalance theory is the most common among health care professionals.

Proponents state that because the body does not store enough water for exercise and athletes do not ingest enough water to replace the amounts they lose during exercise, EAMC are the result of fluid and electrolyte depletion, which results in the sensitization of select nerve terminals. The resulting contracture of the interstitial space increases the mechanical pressure on select motor nerve endings and finally results in EAMC. Exercise in hot and humid conditions exacerbates the amount of fluid and electrolytes lost, thereby facilitating cramps.

Support for the dehydration–electrolyte imbalance theory comes mainly from research classified as level 4 and 5 evidence. Miners develop cramps because of their sweat losses while working in hot and humid conditions. More recently, researchers observed that the majority of cramping (95%, 87 of 92) occurred in hot months—specifically, when football players exercised in environmental conditions in which the risk of developing heat illness was "high" or "extreme." Other evidence for this theory comes from case studies and other observational work in which large sweat losses occurred in exercising athletes. Some health professionals postulate that sweat glands are unable to reabsorb sodium at "high" sweat rates. The prevailing belief is that EAMC are a warning sign of dehydration–electrolyte imbalance.

The dehydration–electrolyte imbalance theory does not, however, explain EAMC in athletes exercising in cool, temperature-controlled environments. For example, Maughan reported that marathoners (18%, 15 of 82) still developed EAMC even though the ambient temperature was 10 to 12°C. Thus, it is unlikely that a hot and humid environment is required for the development of EAMC, although they may occur more frequently under conditions of elevated ambient temperatures.

Regarding fluid losses in crampers and noncrampers, plasma volume losses in runners with EAMC (5.2%) were not significantly different from those of runners without EAMC (4.4%), nor were losses in blood volume (1.7% vs 1.3%) or body weight. Moreover, sweat rate and sodium/fluid losses are often not different in athletes who develop EAMC. Finally, a correlation between body weight losses and EAMC has not been established in several groups of athletes.

The treatment for EAMC also fails to support the dehydration–electrolyte imbalance theory. If EAMC were due to dehydration, the simple cure would be fluid replacement. However, when carbohydrate-electrolyte fluids were ingested at a rate that matched sweat loss, EAMC still occurred in 69% of athletes (9 of 13). Moreover, athletes who develop EAMC often ingest similar amounts of fluid during exercise as do their noncramping counterparts. Oral fluid ingestion may be ineffective, and intravenous fluid may provide a faster delivery for athletes suffering from acute EAMC. It is interesting that stretching the affected muscle almost immediately relieves EAMC and yet has no effect on the fluid conditions of the body.

Overall, the dehydration–electrolyte imbalance theory has limitations: First, inferences of cause and effect cannot be made from observational data (eg, field studies); causation may be inferred only from meta-analyses and randomized, experimental research designs (evidence levels 1 and 2, respectively). Second, although EAMC may appear in the presence of significant electrolyte and/or fluid losses during exercise, numerous other variables associated with exercise may be factors (eg, accumulation of metabolites, intensity of exercise, and acclimatization). Because athletes who experience EAMC often have significant fluid deficits, restoring body fluids is an appropriate precautionary measure against the development of more serious forms of heat illness (eg, exertional hyponatremia, heat stroke).

The neuromuscular theory of EAMC proposes that muscle overload and neuromuscular fatigue cause an imbalance between excitatory impulses from muscle spindles and inhibitory impulses from Golgi tendon organs (GTOs). These localized EAMC tend to occur when the muscle is contracting in an already-shortened position. The reduced tension in the muscle tendon likely reduces the inhibitory feedback from GTO afferents, thereby predisposing the muscle to cramp from the imbalance between inhibitory and excitatory drives to the alpha motor neuron. This enhanced excitability at the spinal level results in an increase in alpha motor neuron discharge to the muscle fibers, producing a localized muscle cramp.

Study designs that examine the plausibility of the neuromuscular system's role in EAMC are stronger than those for dehydration (levels 3 to 5): animal, exercising humans, and stretching for EAMC. These varying models and treatment observations are more consistent with the neuromuscular theory than with the dehydration–electrolyte imbalance theory.

In felines, muscle spindle and GTO activity were measured following neuromuscular fatigue induced by supramaximal stimulation (100 Hz). Fifty percent of type Ia (25 of 49) and 55% of IIa (18 of 33) muscle spindle afferents increased their resting discharge following fatiguing electrical stimulation. Similarly, feline GTO discharge rate was lowered and delayed with fatigue induced with a similar protocol. Thus, neuromuscular fatigue appeared to decrease the inhibition from the GTO and increase the excitatory stimuli from muscle spindles. These effects may result in a heightened excitatory state at the spinal level.

In humans, EAMC occurs more frequently at the end of competitions and physical work and when the muscle contracts while it is already shortened. Stretching, the primary treatment for acute EAMC, is thought to relieve EAMC via autogenic inhibition. Stretching increases the tension in the muscle's tendon, resulting in GTO activation and an increase in inhibition of the alpha motor neuron, which may restore the physiological relationship between excitatory and inhibitory impulses to the alpha motor neuron.

The neuromuscular theory also has limitations. The report of altered muscle spindle and GTO activity relies on difficult methodologies that have produced inconsistent results. The majority of GTO Ib afferents (5 of 8, 63%) have only a slight decline or no change in firing in response to stretching of a fatigued muscle. Neuromuscular fatigue often induces muscle afferent fatigue with supramaximal electrical stimulation (eg, 100 Hz). Normal human muscle recruitment patterns indicate stimulation frequencies much lower (eg, < 30 Hz) than those used to induce fatigue in animal studies (eg, 100 Hz). Low electrical stimulation frequencies closer to normal recruitment patterns (eg, 16 to 32 Hz) have successfully induced cramps in humans. Thus, the frequencies used to support the neuromuscular theory do not match normal neuromuscular signaling in humans. Finally, it is unclear how fatigued a muscle needs to become for an EAMC to occur or whether the neuromuscular fatigue is occurring peripherally (ie, in the muscle) and/or centrally (in the spinal cord or brain). Moreover, it is unlikely that neuromuscular fatigue induced with electrical stimulation is the same as fatigue induced with volitional muscle contractions, given that larger diameter motor neurons/units are stimulated first with electrical stimulation and last with volitional contractions. Muscle fatigue is a continuum rather than an absolute condition. It is likely that the degree of fatigue required to elicit cramping is unique to each athlete.

Because EAMC occur in a variety of situations, environmental conditions, and populations, it is unlikely that a single factor (eg, dehydration, electrolyte imbalance, or neuromuscular factors) is responsible for causing them directly. It is more likely that EAMC are due to a combination of factors that simultaneously occur under specific physiological circumstances in each athlete.

Treatment of EAMC

The paucity of experimental data regarding the cause of EAMC has led to a plethora of treatments for EAMC, confirming the lack of understanding and consensus for EAMC etiology. Many of these treatment options are anecdotal and unsupported by experimental research: ingesting mustard, pickle juice, sports drinks, cryotherapy, thermotherapy, massage, decreasing exercise intensity, body position, intravenous infusion, and TENS (transcutaneous electric nerve stimulation) therapy.

The dehydration–electrolyte theory suggests that ingesting fluids containing electrolytes is beneficial to treat and alleviate EAMC. However, owing to the minimal amount of electrolytes in many sports drinks, it may be difficult to sufficiently replace the volume of electrolytes lost during exercise even if the athlete has modest sweat losses and sweat sodium content. Assuming that a relationship between dehydration–electrolyte imbalance and EAMC exists, the National Athletic Trainers' Association recommends that athletes prone to muscle cramping add 0.3 to 0.7 g/L of salt to their drinks to stave off muscle cramps. Others have recommended adding higher amounts of sodium (about 3.0 to 6.0 g/L) to sports drinks based on the frequency of EAMC. Note that fluids and electrolytes are not absorbed immediately after ingestion; that is, even hypotonic fluids require at least 13 minutes to be absorbed into the circulatory system. Theoretically, intravenous infusion of fluids removes this delay, and it has been used to aid athletes who develop acute EAMC. However, experimental evidence regarding the effectiveness of intravenous fluid infusion on EAMC is still lacking.

Stretching, quinine, and beta-blockers have stronger levels of evidence (level 2 or 3) to support their use, based on drug trials with human participants and other research. If the athlete has no underlying illness, then the most common treatment for EAMC is stretching, which has proven to be effective for EAMC and other types of muscle cramps but may be ineffective for "heat cramps." Therefore, moderate stretching of the affected muscle to alleviate the cramp is recommended.

Once a cramp is alleviated, health care providers should determine what factors may be involved (eg, diabetes mellitus, thyroid disease).

Prevention of EAMC

Despite the lack of direct evidence, maintaining hydration and adequate electrolyte levels is a good prevention strategy for individuals susceptible to EAMC. Fluid volumes of 1.8 L per hour have been well tolerated by tennis athletes who are susceptible to EAMC. Health professionals should monitor each athlete's fluid losses and recommend replacement during and after exercise (eg, obligatory fluid losses). Monitoring an athlete's body weight is an easy method of ensuring adequate fluid replacement and individualizes each athlete's fluid needs.

An athlete who ingests a liter of water or hypotonic sports drink at least 1 hour before competition can be confident that the majority of the fluid, electrolytes, and nutrients have been absorbed and are available in the body. Fluids should be available and easily accessible throughout practices and competitions. A balanced diet is important given that much of fluid and electrolyte replacement occurs during meals.

A common perception is that level of conditioning is a factor in the development of EAMC. There is a strong theoretical basis for performing exercises that target the neuromuscular system to prevent EAMC. Prevention exercises that target muscle spindle and GTO receptors should be implemented to delay neuromuscular fatigue onset and, hence, EAMC. Plyometric exercises may be beneficial to elicit neural adaptations in muscle spindle and GTO receptor firing, enhancing efficiency and sensitivity of reflexive and descending pathways used for neuromuscular control. Endurance training may also serve as an effective means of preventing EAMC by expanding plasma volume and the extracellular fluid compartment and delaying neuromuscular fatigue.

Dehydration

Vigorous or prolonged physical activity (i.e. during endurance sport or exercise) can lead to an increase in the body's core temperature.

This usually results in a higher sweat rate which leads to the loss of bodily fluids and electrolytes and can cause mild to moderate dehydration.

- Optimal sports performance requires an athlete to be at their peak – physically and mentally.

- When exercising, you lose fluid and electrolytes through sweat which can cause dehydration.

- Dehydration can affect your mental and physical state, leading to problems that affect your performance, such as:

   ◦ Cramps, spasms, and soreness

   ◦ Fatigue

   ◦ Impaired concentration

Relieving Dehydration During Sports and Exercise

When preventing and relieving dehydration related to sports and exercise, it is important to replace both the lost fluid and electrolytes. You need electrolytes for two key reasons:

- To retain the fluid you consume

- To help with nerve and muscle function

Hydralyte is an electrolyte solution clinically formulated for rapid rehydration that is suitable for athletes of all ages. It is low in sugar and high in the electrolytes lost in sweat, which your body needs to perform at its best. Athletes are required to perform at optimal levels, staying hydrated is a big factor in overall performance.

Exercise-related Heat Exhaustion

Heat-related illness can affect you as heat cramps, heat exhaustion, or heat stroke.

Exercise-related heat exhaustion is an illness caused by getting too hot when you exercise. During heat exhaustion, the body temperature rises above normal.

The brain usually keeps the body temperature within a degree or two of 98.6 °F (37 °C). This temperature control is important because many processes in the body only work well within a certain range of temperatures.

The body has several ways to lower the body temperature when it gets too high. the body can cool itself by sweating. When sweat evaporates, it lowers the temperature. The body can also lower the temperature by sending more blood to the skin and to the arms, legs, and head. This lets more heat can escape. If the body cannot get rid of the extra heat, the body temperature will rise. In heat exhaustion, the body temperature may rise to 101 °F (38.3 °C) to 104 °F (40 °C). This can make you feel weak and dizzy. The heart may not be able to pump enough blood. This can make you collapse.

Heat exhaustion is less serious than heat stroke, another heat-related illness. But heat exhaustion can lead to heat stroke if it is not treated. In heat stroke, the body temperature rises even higher. This stops basic processes in the body. This can cause serious problems, including death.

Unfortunately, heat exhaustion is common. In the U.S., exercise-related heat exhaustion is a common problem in athletes, especially football players. It is also common in military recruits in basic training.

What Causes Exercise-related Heat Exhaustion?

Exercise-related heat exhaustion happens when the body can no longer get rid of the extra heat made during exercise, and the body temperature rises more than is healthy. Not drinking enough fluids during exercise can also cause dehydration. Together, these things can make you collapse.

Exercising outdoors on a hot day can cause heat exhaustion. But humidity also plays a large role. In high humidity, the body can't use sweat to cool itself. This robs the body of one of the most important ways of getting rid of extra heat.

Many other things can make it harder for the body to get rid of extra heat. These include:

- Being in poor physical shape.
- Having an infection.
- Being dehydrated.
- Using alcohol before exercising.

- Being obese.

- Not being used to a hot environment.

- Taking certain medicines such as stimulants, antihistamines, and medicines for epilepsy.

- Having certain medical conditions, like sickle cell disease or conditions that decrease sweat.

- Having a chronic illness.

Adults over the age of 65 and young children also have a higher risk for heat exhaustion and other heat-related illnesses. This is because their bodies cannot cool down as easily as those of older children and younger adults.

Who is at Risk for Heat Exhaustion?

These groups may be more likely to get heat exhaustion when exercising in hot, humid conditions:

- Women.

- People of white background.

- People who grew up in more temperate climates.

What are the Symptoms of Heat Exhaustion?

The main symptom of heat exhaustion is a body temperature of 101°F (38.3°C) to 104°F (40°C). Some symptoms may be warning signs that heat exhaustion is about to happen. Symptoms may vary depending on the how serious the heat exhaustion is. Signs and symptoms may include:

- Rapid heartbeat,

- Fast breathing,

- Heavy sweating,

- Dizziness,

- Fainting,

- Nausea, vomiting, or diarrhea,

- Headache,

- Weakness,

- Muscle cramps,

- Mild, temporary confusion,

- Low blood pressure,

- Persistent fatigue, different from just being tired from a hard training session, occurs when fatigue continues even after adequate rest.

- Elevated resting heart rate, a persistently high heart rate after adequate rest such as in the morning after sleep, can be an indicator of overtraining.

- Reduced heart rate variability.

- Increased susceptibility to infections.

- Increased incidence of injuries.

- Irritability.

- Depression.

- Mental breakdown.

- Burnout.

It is important to note the difference between overtraining and over-reaching; over-reaching is when an athlete is undergoing hard training but with adequate recovery, overtraining however, is when an athlete is undergoing hard training without the adequate recovery. With over-reaching, the consequential drop in performance can be resolved in a few days or weeks.

Performance

- Early onset of fatigue.

- Decreased aerobic capacity (VO_2 max).

- Poor physical performance.

- Inability to complete workouts.

- Delayed recovery.

It is also important to remember that the effect of overtraining is not isolated only to affecting the athlete's athletic ability but it can have implications on other areas of life such as performance in studies or the work force. An overtrained athlete who is suffering from physical and or psychological symptoms could also have trouble socialising with friends and family, studying for an exam or prepping for work.

Cause

Like pharmacological drugs, physical exercise may be chemically addictive. Addiction can be defined as the frequent engaging in the behavior to a greater extent or for a longer time period than intended. It is theorized that this addiction is due to natural endorphins and dopamine generated and regulated by the exercise. Whether strictly due to this chemical by-product or not, some people can be said to become addicted to or fixated on psychological/physical effects of physical exercise and fitness. This may lead to overexercise, resulting in the "overtraining" syndrome.

Mechanism

A number of possible mechanisms for overtraining have been proposed:

- Microtrauma to the muscles are created faster than the body can heal them.

- Amino acids are used up faster than they are supplied in the diet. This is sometimes called "protein deficiency".

- Systemic inflammation which results in the release of cytokines activating an immune response.

Prevention

Preventing overtraining is important for many athletes, who want to avoid taking time off to recover from overtraining. One method preferred by many collegiate and professional level athletes is the incorporation of active recovery into training. The gradual varying of intensity and volume of training is also an effective way to prevent overtraining. The athlete should be closely monitored by keeping records of weight, diet and heart rate and the training program should be adjusted in accordance to different physical and emotional stresses.

Exertional Rhabdomyolysis

Exertional rhabdomyolysis (ER) is the breakdown of muscle from extreme physical exertion. It is one of many types of rhabdomyolysis that can occur, and because of this the exact prevalence and incidence are unclear.

Cause

ER is more likely to occur when strenuous exercise is performed under high temperatures and humidity. Poor hydration levels before, during, and after strenuous bouts of exercise have also been reported to lead to ER. This condition and its signs and symptoms are not well known amongst the sport and fitness community and because of this it is believed that the incidence is greater but highly underreported.

Risks that lead to ER include exercise in hot and humid conditions, improper hydration, inadequate recovery between bouts of exercise, intense physical training, and inadequate fitness levels for beginning high intensity workouts. Dehydration is one of the biggest factors that can give almost immediate feedback from the body by producing very dark-colored urine.

Mechanism

Anatomy

Exertional rhabdomyolysis results from damage to the intercellular proteins inside the sarcolemma. Myosin and actin break down in the sarcomeres when ATP is no longer available due to injury to the sarcoplasmic reticulum. Damage to the sarcolemma and sarcoplasmic reticulum from direct trauma or high force production causes a high influx of calcium into the muscle fibers increasing calcium permeability. Calcium ions build up in the mitochondria, impairing cellular respiration. The mitochondria are unable to produce enough ATP to power the cell properly. Reduction in ATP production impairs the cells ability to extract calcium from the muscle cell.

The ion imbalance causes calcium-dependent enzymes to activate which break down muscle proteins even further. A high concentration of calcium activates muscle cells, causing the muscle to contract while inhibiting its ability to relax.

The increase of sustained muscle contraction leads to oxygen and ATP depletion with prolonged exposure to calcium. The muscle cell membrane pump may become damaged allowing free form myoglobin to leak into the bloodstream.

Physiology

Rhabdomyolysis causes the myosin and actin to degenerate into smaller proteins that travel into the circulatory system. The body reacts by increasing intracellular swelling to the injured tissue to send repair cells to the area. This allows creatine kinase and myoglobin to be flushed from the tissue where it travels in the blood until reaching the kidneys. In addition to the proteins released, large quantities of ions such as intracellular potassium, sodium, and chloride find their way into the circulatory system. Intracellular potassium ion has deleterious effects on the heart's ability to generate action potentials leading to cardiac arrhythmias. Consequently, this can affect peripheral and central perfusion which in turn can affect all major organ systems in the body.

When the protein reaches the kidneys it causes a strain on the anatomical structures reducing its effectiveness as a filter for the body. The protein acts like a dam as it forms into tight aggregates when it enters the renal tubules. In addition, the increased intracellular calcium has greater time to bind due to the blockage allowing for renal calculi to form. As a result this causes urine output to decrease allowing for the uric acid to build up inside the organ. The increased acid concentration allows the iron from the aggregate protein to be released into the surrounding renal tissue. Iron then strips away molecular bonds of the surrounding tissue which eventually will lead to kidney failure if the tissue damage is too great.

Mechanical Consideration

Muscle degeneration from rhabdomyolysis destroys the myosin and actin filaments in the affected tissue. This initiates the body's natural reaction to increase perfusion to the area allowing for an influx of specialized cells to repair the injury. However, the swelling increases the intracellular pressure beyond normal limits. As the pressure builds in the muscle tissue, the surrounding tissue is crushed against underlying tissue and bone. This is known as compartment syndrome which leads to greater death of the surrounding muscle tissue around the injury. As the muscle dies this will cause pain to radiate from the affected area into the compartmentalized tissue. A loss of range of motion from swelling will also be seen in the affected limb. Along with muscle strength weakness associated with the muscles involved from loss of filament interaction.

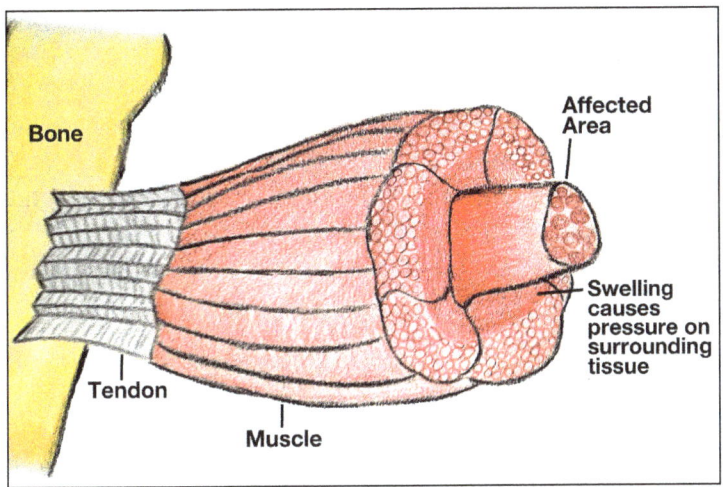

Compartment syndrome in muscle.

Dehydration is a common risk factor for exertional rhabdomyolsis because it causes a reduction of plasma volume during exertion. This leads to a reduction of blood flow through the vascular system which inhibits blood vessel constriction.

Diagnosis

Exertional rhabdomyolysis, the exercise-induced muscle breakdown that results in muscle pain/soreness, is commonly diagnosed using the urine myoglobin test accompanied by high levels of creatine kinase (CK). Myoglobin is the protein released into the bloodstream when skeletal muscle is broken down. The urine test simply examines whether myoglobin is present or absent. When results are positive the urine normally obtains a dark, brown color followed by serum CK level evaluation to determine the severity of muscle damage. Elevated levels of serum CK greater than 5,000 U/L that are not caused by myocardial infarction, brain injury, or disease generally indicate serious muscle damage confirming diagnosis of ER.

Prevention

Military data suggest that the risk of exertional rhabdomyolysis can be lowered by engaging in prolonged lower-intensity exercise, as opposed to high-intensity exercise over a shorter time period. In all athletic programs, three features should be present: (1) emphasizing prolonged lower-intensity exercise, as opposed to repetitive max intensity exercises; (2) adequate rest periods and a high-carbohydrate diet, to replenish glycogen stores; and (3) proper hydration, to enhance renal clearance of myoglobin. Also, exercise in above-average temperature and humidity can increase risk for ER. ER can be avoided by gradually increasing intensity during new exercise regimens, properly hydrating, acclimatization, and avoidance of diuretics during times of strenuous activity.

Treatment

After ER is diagnosed, treatment is applied to 1) avoid renal dysfunction and 2) alleviate symptoms. This should be followed by recommended rehabilitation program, exercise prescription (ExRx). Treatment involves extensive hydration normally done through IV fluid replacement with administration of normal saline until CK levels reduce to a maximum of 1,000 U/L. Proper treatment will ensure hydration and normalize muscle discomfort (pain), flu-like symptoms, CK levels, and myoglobin levels for patient to begin ExRx.

Although sufficient evidence is currently lacking, supplementation with a combination of sodium bicarbonate and mannitol is commonly utilized to prevent kidney failure in rhabdomyolysis patients. Sodium bicarbonate alkalizes urine to stop myoglobin from precipitating in renal tubules. Mannitol has several effects, including vasodilatation of renal vasculature, osmotic diuresis, and free-radical scavenging.

Recovery

Before initiating any form of physical activity, the individual must demonstrate a normal level of functioning with all previous symptoms absent. Physical activity should be supervised by a health care professional in case of a recurrence. However, in some low risk individuals, supervision by a medical professional is not required as long as individual follows up with weekly checkups. Proper hydration prior to performing physical activity and performing exercise in cool, dry environments may reduce the chances of developing a reoccurring episode of ER. Lastly, it is imperative for urine and blood values to be monitored along with careful observation for redevelopment of any signs or symptoms.

The recovery program focuses on progressively conditioning/reconditioning the individual and improving functional mobility. However, special considerations prior to participating in rehabilitation program include the individual's 1) extent of muscle injury, if any 2) level of fitness before incident and 3) weight training experience. These special considerations collectively are a form of assessing the individual's capacity to perform physical activity, which is ultimately used to specify the ExRx design.

Sports Injury

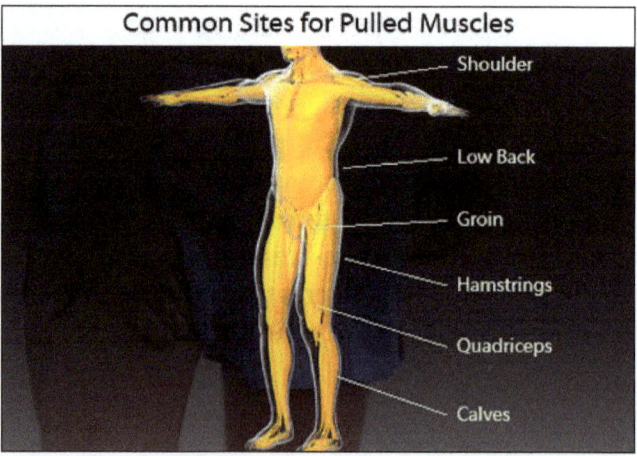

Sports injuries are injuries that occur when engaging in sports or exercise. Sports injuries can occur due to overtraining, lack of conditioning, and improper form or technique. Failing to warm up increases the risk of sports injuries. Bruises, strains, sprains, tears, and broken bones can result from sports injuries. Soft tissues like muscles, ligaments, tendons, fascia, and bursae may be affected. Traumatic brain injury (TBI) is another potential type of sports injury.

Pulled Muscle

Muscle strain is another name for a pulled muscle. It occurs when a muscle is overstretched and tears. Symptoms of a pulled muscle may include pain, swelling, weakness, and difficulty or inability to use the muscle. Muscles in the quadriceps, the calves, hamstrings, groin, low back, and shoulder are the most common sites for pulled muscles. Minor muscle strains resolve with RICE -- Rest, Ice, Compression, and Elevation. Nonsteroidal anti-inflammatory drugs (NSAIDs) may help manage pain and swelling as well. More serious muscle strains require evaluation and treatment by a doctor.

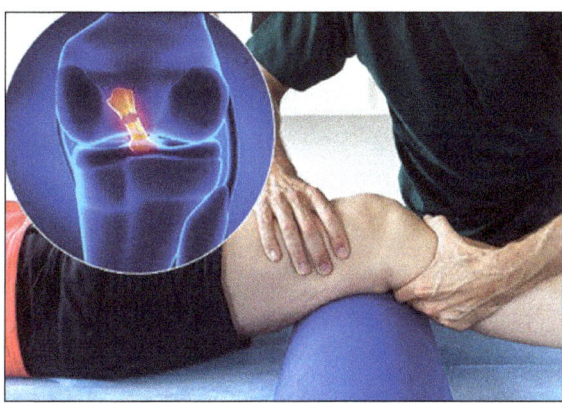

Torn ACL

The anterior cruciate ligament (ACL) helps hold the knee joint together and provides stability. A torn ACL is a sports injury that may occur when landing the wrong way, changing direction or stopping quickly, or from a direct blow to the knee. People who suffer a torn ACL may hear a pop and then feel their knee no longer functions. Pain, swelling, and loss of range of motion are symptoms of a torn ACL. It may be difficult to walk. A torn ACL needs to be reconstructed surgically, usually using a graft from another ligament in the patient's own body. Significant rehabilitation is necessary to restore the strength and function of the knee joint after surgery. Depending on the age, health status, and desired activity level of the patient, some may not elect to have surgery. In that case, braces and physical therapy will not cure the condition, but may provide some relief.

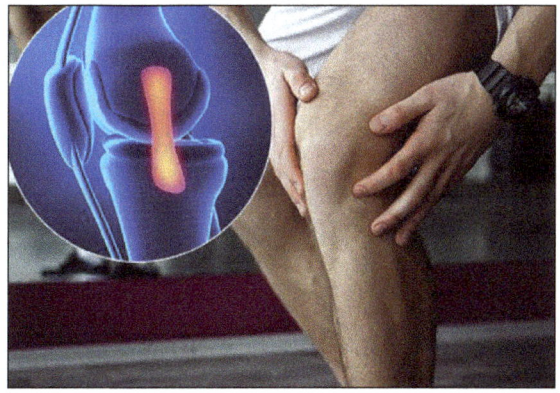

Torn MCL

The medial collateral ligament (MCL) connects the upper leg bone (femur) to the larger bone of the lower leg (tibia). It is located on the inner side of the knee. The MCL is typically injured when the knee joint is pushed sideways when making a wrong move or by receiving a direct blow to the knee. A torn MCL results in pain, swelling, and instability of the joint. The condition is often treated with ice, bracing, and physical therapy. If other structures in the knee are injured or if the torn MCL is severe, surgery may be recommended.

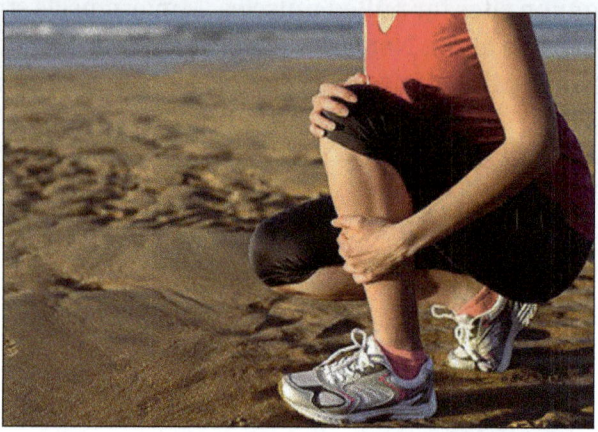

Shin Splints

Shin splints are throbbing, aching, or stabbing pain on the insides of the lower leg. Shin splints are a repetitive use injury that may occur in runners or those who are beginning to exercise. Pain occurs when muscles and tendons around the tibia (the larger of the two lower leg bones) become inflamed. Stretching, resting, and applying ice can help relieve shin splints. Nonsteroidal anti-inflammatory drugs (NSAIDs) can reduce pain and swelling. Bandaging the area may help prevent swelling. Flat feet increase the risk of shin splints. Orthotics and proper athletic shoes may offer support and decrease the risk of shin splints.

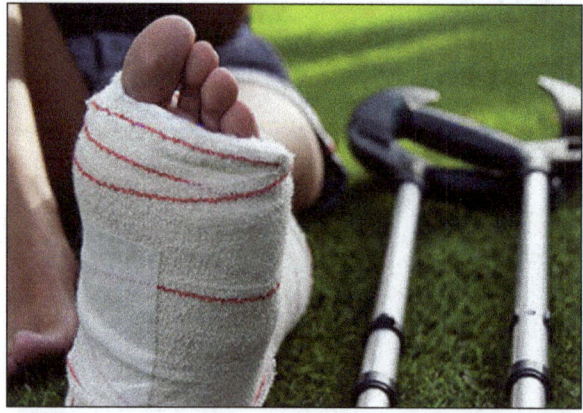

Stress Fracture

A stress fracture is an overuse injury that occurs when muscles are no longer able to absorb the impact from physical activity, and a bone absorbs the pressure, resulting in a break. Stress fractures can occur when increasing activity, especially too quickly. The majority of stress fractures occur in the lower legs and feet. Women are more prone to stress fractures than men. Stress fractures cause pain with activity. Rest is prescribed to allow a stress fracture to heal. Sometimes a special shoe or a brace helps decrease stress on the bone, which facilitates healing.

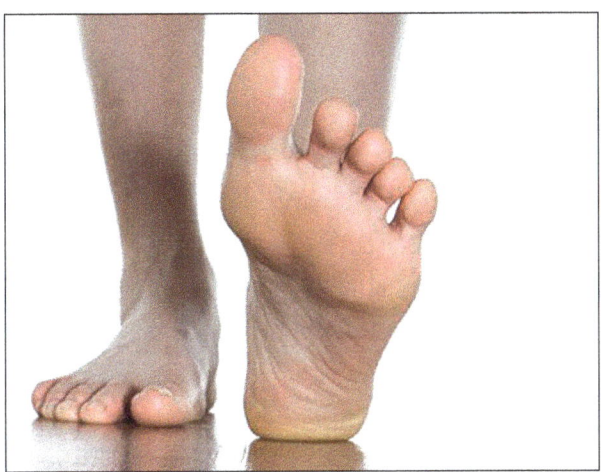

Plantar Fasciitis

The plantar fascia is a ligament that connects the heel to the front of the foot, supporting the arch. Plantar fasciitis is inflammation of this ligament. It causes heel pain often felt the first thing in the morning after getting out of bed or after being active. Stress and strain on the feet increases the risk of plantar fasciitis. Obesity, tight calf muscles, repetitive use, high arches, and new athletic activities are all risk factors for this condition. Plantar fasciitis is treated with rest, ice, nonsteroidal anti-inflammatory drugs (NSAIDs), and special stretching exercises. Cushioning insoles may provide relief. Wearing splints at night may help decrease pain. More severe cases of plantar fasciitis may be treated with cortisone injections, physical therapy, and surgery.

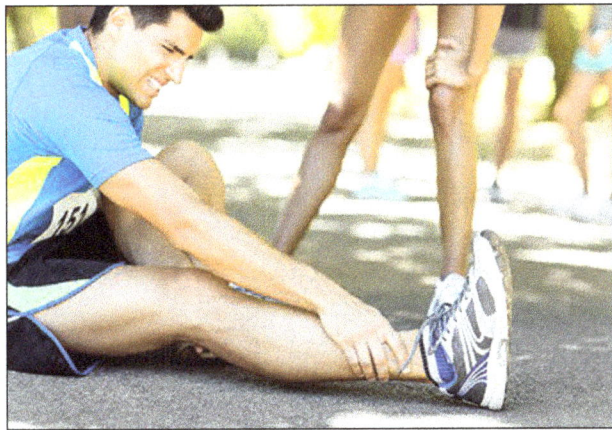

Sprained Ankle

A sprained ankle occurs when the ligaments that support the joint become overstretched. Ankle sprains may occur when playing sports or doing everyday activities. Stepping wrong on an uneven surface or stepping in a way that twists or rolls the foot may lead to an ankle sprain. Sprains and the pain they cause may range from mild to severe. RICE -- rest, ice, compression, and elevation -- are used to treat ankle sprains. Nonsteroidal anti-inflammatory drugs (NSAIDs) can alleviate pain and swelling. Severe sprains may require a brace or cast for several weeks to facilitate healing.

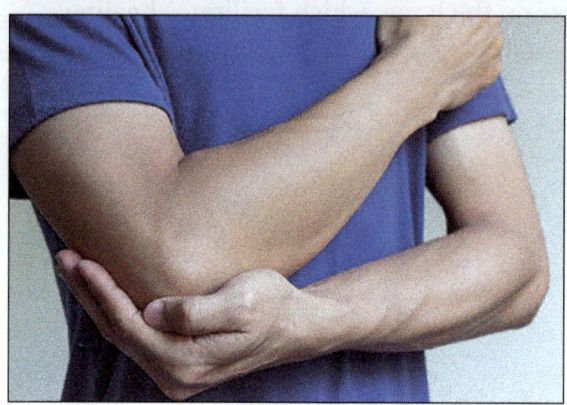

Tennis Elbow

Tennis elbow is an overuse injury that may be associated with playing racket sports. Plumbers, painters and those in similar professions are also at risk. Tennis elbow involves inflammation of the tendons on the outside of the elbow caused by small tears. Tennis elbow causes pain and may be associated with a weak grip. Rest and nonsteroidal anti-inflammatory medications can help alleviate tennis elbow symptoms. Wearing a special brace on the forearm may help decrease pressure on the sore area. Physical therapy may be helpful. Steroid injections can decrease inflammation. Surgery may be an option for tennis elbow when other treatments have failed.

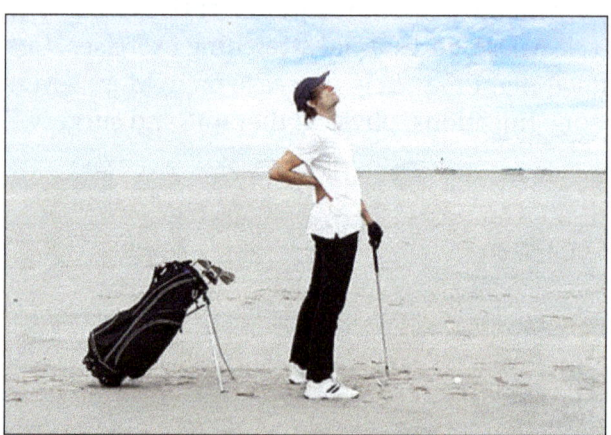

Low Back Pain

There are many causes of low back pain. Back pain may be due to overuse, such as playing one too many rounds of golf or lifting heavy weights. This kind of back strain usually resolves on its own without treatment. Rest and anti-inflammatory medications can provide relief. Using proper form when exercising and increasing the duration of workouts slowly can help protect the back. In some cases, it may be necessary to modify exercise technique or perform daily activities in a different way in order to reduce the risk of back injury. Other causes of back pain may be more serious and require medical or surgical intervention.

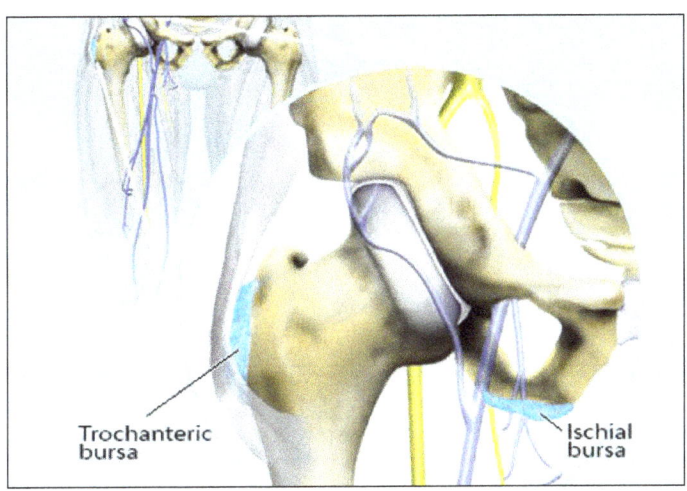

Trochanteric bursa   Ischial bursa

Hip Bursitis

The hip region contains two major bursae. The one located on the outside of the hip is called the trochanteric bursa. The other is called the ischial bursa which covers the ischial tuberosity, more commonly known as the sits bones. Inflammation of either bursae may lead to stiffness and pain around the hip joint not to be confused with the true joint pain of arthritis. Overuse from running, cycling, and similar activities can lead to hip bursitis. The condition causes hip pain that tends to be worse at night. Getting up from a seated position may cause pain. Treatment of hip bursitis consists of avoiding activities that produce symptoms and taking nonsteroidal anti-inflammatory drugs (NSAIDs) to reduce pain and swelling. Physical therapy and steroid injections may be warranted. Using a cane or other assistive device may help take the load off the inflamed joint.

References

- Ashley, Linda. Essential Guide to Dance. 2nd ed. London: Hodder & Stoughton, 2004. Print. ISBN 978-0340803202

- How much physical activity do adults need?". Centers for Disease Control and Prevention. 1 December 2011. Retrieved 29 April 2013

- Exercise, causes-of-dehydration, dehydration: hydralyte.ca, Retrieved 14 July, 2019

- Alberts, David S. And Hess, Lisa M. (2005). Fundamentals of Cancer Prevention. Berlin: Springer, ISBN 364238983X

- Benefits of Physical Activity". Centers for Disease Control and Prevention. 6 March 2018. Retrieved 30 April 2018

- Baechle, Thomas R.; Earle, Roger W., eds. (2008). Essentials of strength training and conditioning (3rd ed.). Champaign, IL: Human Kinetics. ISBN 978-0-7360-5803-2.[page needed]

- Sports-injuries: onhealth.com, Retrieved 11 January, 2019

- Walker, Brad. "Overtraining - Learn how to identify Overtraining Syndrome". Stretchcoach.com. Retrieved 2016-05-17

6

Diverse Aspects of Exercise Physiology

The diverse aspects of exercise physiology can be classified as lactace threshold, physical literacy, strength training, exercise intolerance, metabolic equivalent of task (MET), etc. The topics elaborated in this chapter will help in gaining a better perspective about these aspects of exercise physiology.

Exercise as Medicine

Overweightness and obesity are the biggest health problem faced in the twenty-first century. The major causes of this problem are lack of physical activity and excessive consumption of processed food. Individuals who are overweight typically show abnormal cardiovascular function, and obesity is an independent risk factor for cardiovascular diseases, such as hypertension, heart disease, and type 2 diabetes. Hypertension has been found to occur more frequently in overweight compared to lean individuals and poses a risk for hypertension development in young overweight adults. Obesity has also been found to be associated with reduced life expectancy and sudden death largely through its negative effect on the cardiovascular system. Degradation of a number of key autonomic cardiovascular markers, such as reduced heart rate variability and baroreflex sensitivity, is associated with the development of these lifestyle diseases. Also alterations in the metabolic profile, such as dyslipidemia and hyperglycemia, can lead to impairment in cardiac structure and function. Regular exercise has been widely used as preventative medicine to reverse autonomic, cardiovascular, and metabolic decline. Thus, incorporating regular exercise into daily activity may prevent the development of these cardiovascular diseases and accompanying risk factors.

Physical inactivity has been shown to affect health by increasing cardiovascular and metabolic dysfunction. More and more people including children and adolescents are leading a sedentary lifestyle, which leads to a number of health problems. Overweightness and obesity are often accompanied by a lack of physical activity that can lead to more serious health problems, such as metabolic syndrome, type 2 diabetes, and hypertension. Lack of physical activity has also been found to be a major cause of morbidity and mortality. Overweight and obese individuals typically show abnormal cardiovascular function, and obesity has been found to be an independent risk factor for cardiovascular diseases, such as hypertension, type 2 diabetes, and cardiac complications (i.e., heart failure, heart disease). Obesity is associated with reduced life expectancy and sudden death through its negative effect on the cardiovascular system. Overweight and obese individuals usually develop hypertension. Compared to normal weight individuals, overweightness and obesity pose a potential risk for hypertension development in overweight individuals. It was found that a 10 kg excess in weight was associated with a 3 mmHg higher systolic and a 2–3 mmHg higher resting diastolic blood pressure. This can be translated into an estimated increased risk for coronary heart disease of 12% and an increased risk of stroke of 24%. Alterations in the metabolic profile that are commonly found in overweight and obese individuals, such as dyslipidemia and hyperglycemia, can also lead to impairment in cardiac structure and function as adipose tissue accumulates. It has been shown that left ventricular (LV) function and the ratio of the stroke index and LV end-diastolic pressure are reduced with overweightness and obesity. These changes show that depressed LV function has already occurred even in young overweight and obese individuals.

Overwhelming evidence indicates that regular physical activity in the form of both acute and regular aerobic exercise reduces the severity and occurrence of diseases related to unhealthy lifestyles. One single bout of acute exercise has been found to improve vascular function even in normotensive young healthy individuals with a family history of hypertension. Whereas regular aerobic exercise has been shown to improve physical fitness (cardiorespiratory fitness) in addition to improving vascular function. Having high levels of physical fitness, assessed through a sub-maximal or maximal oxygen uptake test, is desirable as low cardiorespiratory fitness has been found to significantly increase the risk of cardiovascular diseases and mortality more so than other factors, such as hypertension, type 2 diabetes, and smoking, and regardless of body mass index. High-intensity interval training (HIIT) is a form of interval sprinting exercise typically performed on a stationary bike and has also been found to improve cardiac and metabolic health of young overweight males and females. Physical activity is so important that failure to lead a physically active lifestyle can result in several abnormalities such as high blood pressure, metabolic syndrome, and type 2 diabetes. Baroreceptor sensitivity (BRS) has also been found to decrease with age, being hypertensive and being overweight and obese.

Overall, regular exercise results in improvement of the pathogenesis and symptoms of specific conditions that include chronic heart failure, coronary heart disease, dyslipidemia, hypertension, insulin resistance, intermittent claudication, obesity, and type 2 diabetes. Other health benefits of regular aerobic exercise include improvement in balance, cognitive functioning, life expectancy, and overall quality of life. The beneficial effects of regular aerobic exercise have been well known. Thus, modification of a sedentary lifestyle by incorporating regular exercise is paramount for maintaining and improving health. Exercise is a powerful stimulus and can reduce the severity of several conditions with its effects being similar to many drug therapies. In this regard, exercise has now been widely accepted as medicine.

Cardiovascular Problems Associated with Physical Inactivity

A sedentary lifestyle, which is associated with overweightness and obesity, typically leads to an increased risk of cardiovascular disease. Currently, overweightness and obesity have been escalating at an alarming rate worldwide. Based on the World Health Organization (WHO, Global Health Observatory data) region data from 2010 to 2014, the prevalence of overweightness and obesity for both males and females at the age of ≥18 years has significantly increased. Women were more likely to be obese than men in 2014 in all WHO regions. Increased numbers of overweight and obese individuals put tremendous pressure and burden on healthcare providers and threatens world health in many countries. Approximately 20–30% of adults worldwide are categorized as clinically obese and numbers are progressively increasing. It has been well established that both high body mass index and a sedentary lifestyle are associated with greater risk of cardiovascular disease.

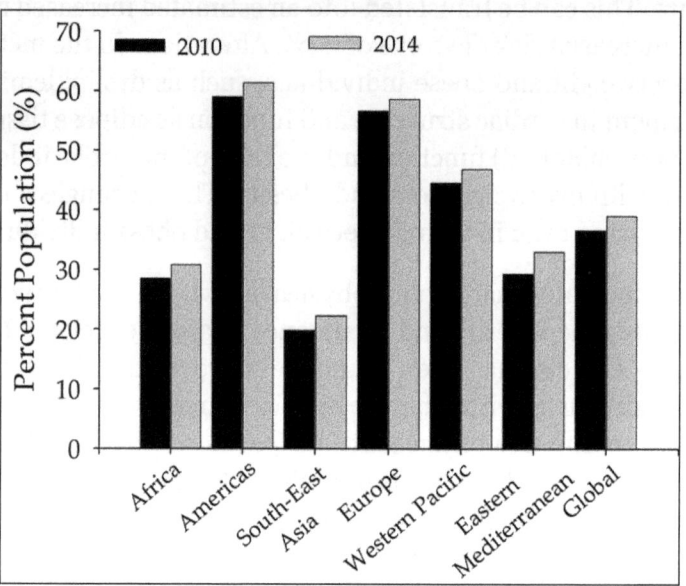

Prevalence of overweight based on WHO region for both sexes.

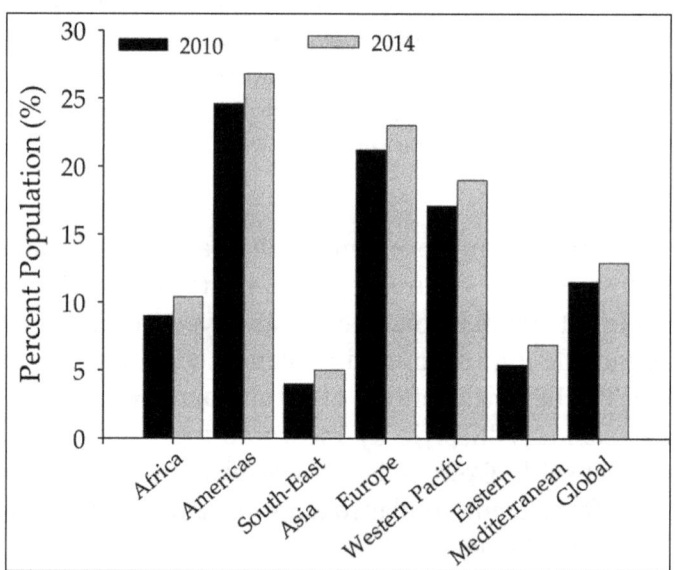

Prevalence of obesity based on the WHO region for both sexes.

It has been shown that overweightness and obesity are accompanied by a cluster of cardiovascular risk factors, which is termed metabolic syndrome and includes hypertension, glucose intolerance, hypertriglyceridemia, and visceral obesity. These conditions occur in approximately one out of four adults over the age of 40. The metabolic syndrome is also associated with insulin resistance and endothelial dysfunction. It is believed that in child obesity, as fat mass increases, insulin resistance develops, which is a determinant of impaired metabolic function at early age. Other health problems accompanying overweightness and obesity include cardiac autonomic dysfunction and endothelial dysfunction. Aberrant cardiac autonomic function has been found in obese children and increased adiposity during childhood increases the risk of obesity, type 2 diabetes, and cardiovascular disease in adulthood. Endothelial dysfunction can be defined as inadequate endothelial-mediated vasodilation, which is typically due to a deficiency of endothelial-derived relaxing factor, nitric oxide (NO) synthesis, and/or release. It is believed that NO deficiency is a primary factor linking insulin resistance and endothelial dysfunction. Thus, it is clear that being sedentary results in increased cardiovascular disease risk, aberrant metabolic, cardiac, autonomic, and endothelial function.

Cardiac Autonomic Function

It has been well established that cardiac autonomic dysfunction is associated with conditions, such as overweight, obesity, and type 2 diabetes. The decline of cardiac autonomic function is typically influenced by an accumulation of visceral fat. Lowered autonomic function was also found to be correlated with higher abdominal-to-peripheral body fat distribution measured by dual energy X-ray absorptiometry in both young and old healthy men. These results suggest that visceral obesity contributes to a decline in autonomic function. Also, young individuals with high abdominal adiposity seemed to undergo an early decline and a premature aging of autonomic function. Thus, hypertension and high levels of central adiposity have an unfavorable effect on cardiac autonomic function, which is reflected by impaired heart rate variability (HRV) and baroreflex sensitivity (BRS).

HRV is a marker that is commonly used to assess cardiac autonomic function and can be defined as beat-to-beat variation in the heart rate of individuals possessing normal sinus rhythm. HRV has been shown to be an indicant of healthy cardiac autonomic function as it has been found that reduced HRV predicts increased cardiovascular disease and mortality. High body mass index, which is commonly found in overweight and obese individuals, is also associated with reduced HRV, which contributes to decreased parasympathetic activity and increased sympathetic activity. BRS is another marker of cardiac autonomic function that provides information about the ability to increase parasympathetic or vagal activity and to decrease sympathetic activity in response to sudden increases in blood pressure. BRS, which is typically reduced as people age, is an indicant of the body's autonomic nervous system sensitivity in responding to sudden blood pressure changes. Low BRS is a marker of reduced compliance of the carotid artery. Overweight and obese individuals typically possess endothelial dysfunction that leads to reduced arterial compliance, which is accompanied with a low BRS compared to that of normal weight individuals. Lower BRS has also been found to be associated with high blood pressure, increased sympathetic activity, and diseases related to an unhealthy lifestyle. It seems that low HRV and BRS are affected by the accumulation of visceral fat and metabolic syndrome factors.

Obese children typically have decreased parasympathetic activity compared to normal weight children. It has also been reported that an increased thickness of carotid intima-media in obese children represents a very early sign of atherosclerosis. It has also been found that the earliest signs of atherosclerosis development are lipid deposits in the intimal layer of systemic arteries (aorta), which have been found in children as early as 3 years old and in the coronary arteries of adolescents. Another aberrant change possessed by overweight and obese individuals is high levels of leptin. Several positive correlations among leptin, insulin resistance, and blood pressure existed in overweight children. A reduction in adiposity level, however, brought about a reduction in leptin, which further improved metabolic health, by decreasing insulin, cardiovascular function, and blood pressure. Adiponectin has a major anti-inflammatory and anti-atherogenic effect and has been found to be three times higher in normal weight children compared to overweight and obese children. A 1-year follow-up, following a 1-year intervention, found that children with weight loss had similar adiponectin levels compared to normal weight children. Leptin levels, however, remained higher in overweight and obese children with weight loss. The increase in adiponectin appears to be an early biomarker of improvement in insulin sensitivity. Thus, it is clear that overweightness and obesity in children result in early deposition of fat in the systemic arteries and thickening of arterial walls. These conditions can lead to more serious health complications later in their life if lifestyle modification is not introduced.

Vascular Dysfunction

Overweight and obesity conditions not only result in metabolic dysfunction but also bring about vascular dysfunction. The balance between the ability of the vasculature (arterioles) to vasodilate and vasoconstrict is impaired with the development of overweightness and obesity. The loss of balance between vasodilators and vasoconstrictors is an indicant of endothelial dysfunction. Endothelial dysfunction is now regarded as a precursor of atherogenesis, which further leads to the development of atherosclerosis and diabetic complications. Arterial compliance, and its inverse arterial stiffness, can be defined as the ability of an artery to distend in response to intravascular (transmural) pressure and is commonly termed as stiffening of the arteries. It is well known that overweight and obese individuals typically have high arterial stiffness, and this high arterial stiffness is associated with high body mass index and body fat. Reduction in body mass index, however, has been found to be the strongest determinant of decreased arterial stiffness in severe obese young and middle-aged adults.

Arterial stiffness, which has been considered to be an independent predictor of cardiovascular disease, can be assessed through a reflection wave, commonly known as the augmentation index (AIx) and carotid femoral pulse wave velocity (PWVcf), which is considered to be the gold standard of arterial stiffness assessment. AIx, a reflection wave, is typically assessed by placing an applanation tonometry sensor (e.g., SphygmoCor) on either a radial or carotid artery. AIx then is derived from the ratio of augmented pressure (AP) and pulse pressure (PP), AP/PP. PWVcf is obtained by dividing the distance from the carotid pulse and femoral pulse as measured by a tape measure by the time taken for the arterial pulse to propagate to the carotid and femoral arteries.

Arterial stiffness, which is an indicant of the stiffening of the large arteries, increases with age, especially in central arteries, such as the aorta and carotid artery. Arterial stiffness has also been found to increase with overweightness and obesity, which leads to an increased risk of arteriosclerosis. Overweight and obese children have been found to have high arterial stiffness, assessed through pulse wave velocity. Similar findings were also found in young overweight individuals who had higher arterial stiffness levels compared to the normal weight individuals. Hemodynamic changes accompanying overweightness and obesity include increased arterial wall stress, smooth muscle cell proliferation, thickening of vessel walls, and eventually reduced arterial compliance/increased arterial stiffness. Thickening of vessel walls is likely caused by increased total blood volume and cardiac output to compensate for the metabolic requirements of excess fat. Alterations of hemodynamics, together with other markers of obesity, including chronic inflammation and endothelial dysfunction, have been shown to contribute to the impairment of vasculature structure and function in obese individuals. Thus, the development of arterial stiffness seems to be due to coping mechanisms by the body to meet the metabolic demands caused by excess fat gain. In overweight and obese children, this mechanism seems to develop very early on and carries on until adolescence and adulthood if interventions to reverse this condition are not introduced.

Health Benefits of Aerobic, Interval Sprinting and Resistance Exercise

The health benefits of regular aerobic exercise are well known. Physical activity has been ranked as one of the leading health interventions, which is used to reduce sedentary behavior in children, adolescents, and adults. Currently, exercise guidelines include 150 minutes of exercise per week that consist of moderate and vigorous physical activity combined with resistance training. It has been shown that performing 150 minutes of regular exercise per week results in a reduction of mortality risk by 30% and a decreased risk of diabetes, cancer, depression, and stroke. Despite the positive benefits of regular physical activity, however, many people do not comply with the minimum exercise requirements to maintain health. Lack of motivation and time constrains are possibly the underlying reasons of not performing regular exercise. The importance of regular physical activity is so overwhelming that exercise now has been regarded as medicine.

Exercise has been widely used as preventative medicine to reduce the risk and incidence of cardiovascular and metabolic diseases related to sedentary and unhealthy living. Regular exercise has been shown to improve health and reduce the severity of diseases accompanying an unhealthy lifestyle. The benefits of exercise are overwhelming, and it has been shown that exercise can be used therapeutically for conditions, such as hypertension and insulin resistance, dyslipidemia, type 2 diabetes, obesity, and endothelial dysfunction. Exercise can also be used to improve cardiovascular and metabolic dysfunction that includes enhancing adipokine, cardiometabolic, and other clinical markers. Thus, it is clear that exercise can be used as therapeutic or preventive medicine in order to alleviate lifestyle diseases.

The types of exercise used in past research include aerobic exercise (continuous walking, jogging, and cycling), high-intensity interval training (HIIT), and resistance training (e.g., weights). A study showed that either supervised or unsupervised aerobic exercise resulted in a reduction of body mass index in overweight and obese adolescents. Whereas, other studies have shown that moderate endurance training and interval sprinting exercise have a positive effect on HRV. Both HIIT and aerobic training have been used to induce improvement in HRV in different populations, such as young overweight individuals, type 2 diabetic patients, and older adults. Twenty minutes of HIIT on a stationary cycle ergometer, proceeded with 5 minutes of warm-up and 5 minutes of cool-down, three times per week, for 12 weeks have been found to improve parasympathetic activity in young overweight males.

A study examining type 2 diabetic individuals has also found similar results when 30 minutes, four times per week for 12 weeks of HIIT training on a treadmill resulted in improvement in HRV by 19%. This form of exercise consisted of 3 minutes of warm-up, 6×2 minutes of high intensity at 80–90% of heart rate maximum, separated by 6 minutes of moderate intensity at 50–60% of heart rate maximum with 2-minute recovery intervals, and 3 minutes of cool-down. The improvement of HRV in type 2 diabetes is significant as exercise could potentially prevent type 2 diabetic patients progressing to a condition called diabetic neuropathy later in life. Another HIIT study also showed that HRV was significantly improved in older individuals, whose average age was 74 years, following 14 weeks of cycle ergometer HIIT exercise. Thus, both continuous aerobic exercise and HIIT had positive effects on autonomic function by increasing HRV levels. However, HIIT is currently regarded as a type of exercise that is superior to a typical continuous moderate intensity of aerobic exercise in terms of time efficiency and clinical benefits. The effectiveness of HIIT has been well established in youth and in overweight adult men and women. Twelve weeks of HIIT have shown to improve cardiovascular function, physical fitness, assessed through a maximal oxygen uptake test, and body composition in young overweight women. It seems that both continuous steady state aerobic exercise and HIIT are beneficial for health.

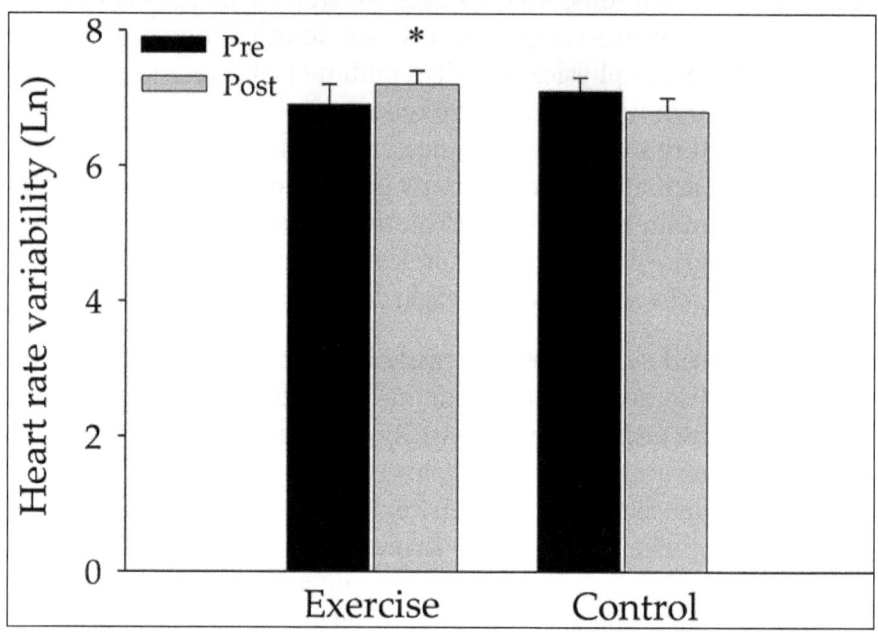

Heart rate variability of overweight young males at pre and post 12 weeks of interval sprinting exercise. *Significant difference between groups, P<0.05.

Modification of HIIT protocols, however, may be needed to suit different populations. For example, HIIT to induce athlete performance would be different with the HIIT used to induce cardiovascular health in healthy sedentary or diseased individuals. Certain exercise effects or adaptations that occur following HIIT training may not occur or be apparent after regular aerobic exercise. Depending on health markers and conditions examined, the magnitude of change following aerobic exercise may be smaller than that of HIIT. For example, it has been demonstrated that arterial stiffness, assessed through PWV and autonomic function are normalized following HIIT in hypertensive individuals, but not following continuous moderate exercise. With HIIT training, the exercise drop-out rate was found to be less compared to continuous steady state aerobic exercise. HIIT is also deemed to be superior in terms of improvement in cardiovascular health compared to regular aerobic exercise. Thus, HIIT may be needed to be incorporated into daily life to induce extra health benefits. HIIT defined as repeated bouts of high-intensity exercise interspersed by rest for 20–30 minutes has also been used to prevent or to reduce severity of diseases related to unhealthy lifestyles. HIIT has been found to improve cardiac and metabolic health of young overweight males and females. The AIx was found to be reduced by 4%, whereas PWVcf velocity was also reduced by 0.4 m.s^{-1} following 12 weeks of HIIT in young overweight males.

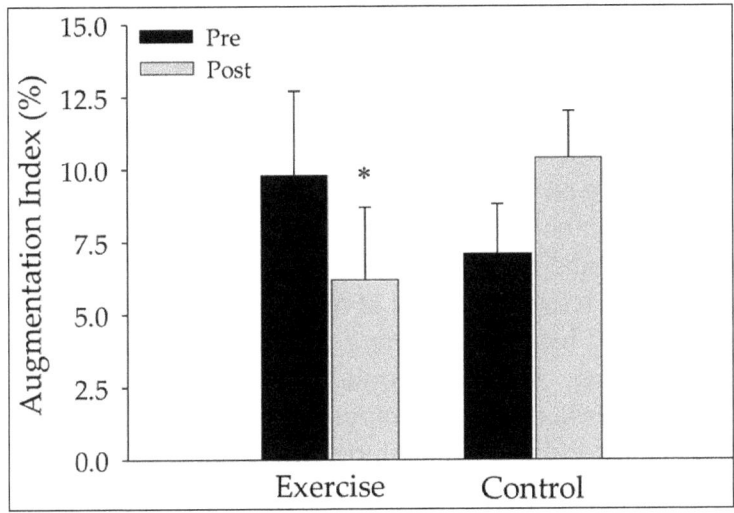

Augmentation index of young overweight males at pre and post 12 weeks of interval sprinting exercise. *Significant difference between groups, P<0.05.

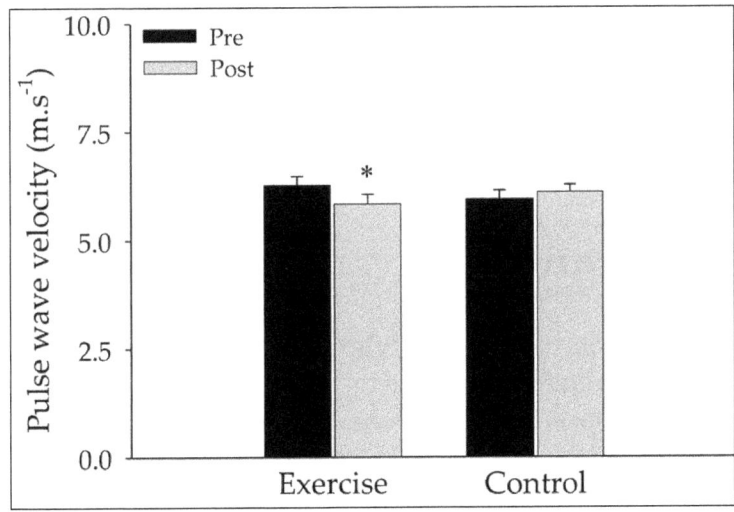

Pulse wave velocity of young overweight males at pre and post 12 weeks of interval sprinting exercise. *Significant difference between groups, P<0.05.

The HIIT employed was an 8-s pedaling sprint at a cadence of 100–120 revolutions per minute (rpm) at 0.5–1 kg of load, followed by a period of lighter intensity exercise at a cadence of 30–40 rpm for 12 seconds, repeated for 20 minutes. Another type of HIIT included cycling on a stationary bike at 80–85% of maximal oxygen uptake for 4 minutes with 5-minute rest intervals, repeated six to eight times. HIIT has also been used in a number of clinical studies involving cardiac rehabilitation, chronic obstructive pulmonary disease, and intermittent claudication disease patients. Thus, a range of interval training exercise programs have been employed to improve cardiovascular and metabolic health.

Resistance exercise is another type of exercise that contributes to cardiovascular and metabolic health. Participating in resistance exercise can maintain muscle mass that declines with aging. Acute resistance training has been found to reduce systolic blood pressure by 11 mmHg and mean arterial pressure by 12 mmHg and systolic blood pressure by 13 mmHg and mean arterial pressure by 12 mmHg with 40 and 80% maximum weight, respectively. The mechanisms underlying this reduction in blood pressure following resistance training is thought to be due to an increased blood flow and shear stress that act on vascular endothelial cells. The increased muscle contraction leads to an increased production of nitric oxide, an important vasodilator. It appears that this mechanism occurs independently of the exercise intensity employed.

The effect of resistance training on arterial stiffness, however, is equivocal. A reduction in central (increased arterial stiffness) but not peripheral arterial compliance was found following 4 months of resistance training in young and healthy middle-aged men. However, only brachial artery endothelial function was improved following 1 year of resistance training, but body mass index, body composition, blood lipids, and lean muscle mass improved. A meta-analysis found that young adults had their arterial stiffness elevated from 14.3 to 20.1% following high-intensity resistance training. In contrast, it has been shown that progressive high-intensity resistance training without an increase in training volume did not alter arterial stiffness in young individuals. Interestingly, the association between resistance training and arterial stiffness was not found in middle-aged individuals. Although high-intensity resistance training has been found to increase arterial stiffness by 11.6%, moderate intensity resistance training did not seem to induce the same effect. Another study showed an unexpected finding when improvement in the muscular strength of young individuals was inversely correlated with arterial stiffness. This finding suggests that resistance training attenuates arterial stiffness. Different protocols and populations possibly could have contributed to the variability of results.

Exercise Intolerance

Exercise intolerance is the primary symptom of chronic diastolic heart failure. It is part of the definition of heart failure and is intimately linked to its pathophysiology. Further, exercise intolerance affects the diagnosis and prognosis of heart failure. In addition, understanding the mechanisms of exercise intolerance can lead to developing and testing rationale treatments for heart failure.

Importance of Exercise Intolerance

Heart failure is defined as a syndrome in which cardiac output is insufficient to meet metabolic demands. This implies that insufficient cardiac output will be expressed symptomatically. Heart failure may often manifest by occasional episodes of acute decompensation with overt systemic volume overload and pulmonary edema. However, the primary chronic symptoms in outpatients, even when well compensated and non-edematous, and whether associated with reduced or normal ejection fraction, are exertional fatigue and dyspnea. In addition, these symptoms and other consequences of exercise intolerance are potent determinants of health-related quality of life in heart failure patients. Several investigators have reported that objective measures, and even subjective estimates, of exercise tolerance predictor survival.

Cardiopulmonary exercise testing on a treadmill or a bicycle ergometer provides the most accurate, reliable, and reproducible assessments of exercise tolerance, and yields multiple important outcomes, including METS, exercise time, exercise workload, blood pressure and heart rate responses, and rate-pressure product. Using commercially available instruments that perform automated expired gas analysis, for both concentration and volume, one can assess at both rest and during exercise, simultaneous measures of oxygen consumption (VO_2), carbon dioxide generation, and ventilatory response. Patient effort is an important modifier of data quality, and can itself be assessed simultaneously and objectively by expired gas analysis as the respiratory exchange ratio, and by the somewhat subjective but more easily obtained measures of perceived effort by the Borg scale and percent age-predicted maximal heart rate.

Submaximal exercise is in some ways a more important outcome variable than peak exercise capacity because it is more applicable to everyday life and is relatively effort independent. Submaximal exercise capacity can be assessed as the ventilatory anaerobic threshold by expired gas analysis, using either the Wasserman-Whipp or the V-slope method. Cardiopulmonary exercise testing measurements and expired gas analysis with automated, commercially available instruments provides measure of both peak oxygen consumption and ventilatory anaerobic threshold that are valid and highly reproducible in elderly patients with diastolic as well as systolic heart failure. Another variable provided by these methods, VE/VCO_2 slope, is a strong predictor of survival, independent of VO_2. It is shown that VE/VCO2 slope is abnormalin patients with DHF, though not as abnormal as in those with systolic heart failure

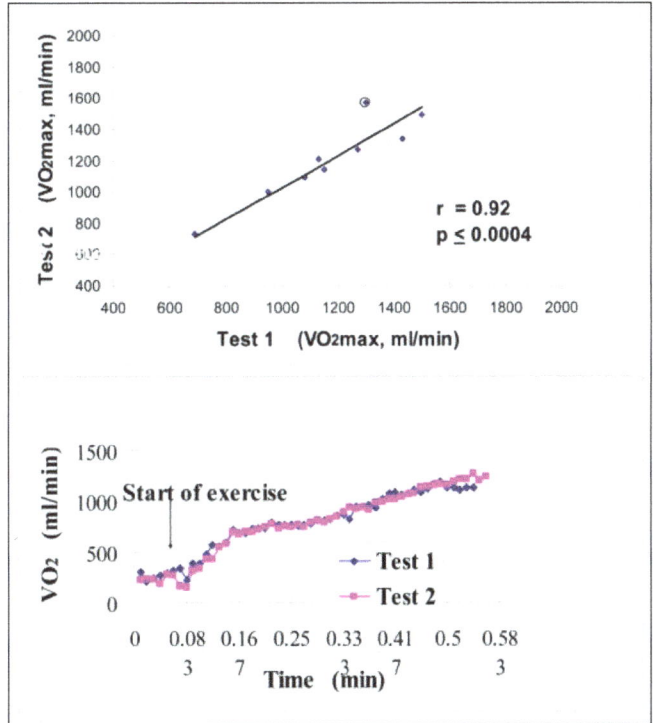

Excellent reproducibility of peak exercise VO_2 in older heart failure patients, including those with LV ejection fraction. Group data shown in top panel; representative patient with 15 second averaged data shown in bottom.

Submaximal exercise performance can also be assessed by timed and distance walk tests. These are simple to perform and are widely available.

Pathophysiology of Exercise Intolerance

In order to understand the pathophysiology of exercise intolerance in DHF, researchers performed a comparative study of maximal exercise testing with expired gas in 119 older subjects in 3 distinct, well-defined groups: heart failure with severe LV systolic dysfunction (mean EF 30%); isolated diastolic heart failure (EF ≥ 50% and no significant coronary, valvular, pericardial, or pulmonary disease and no anemia); and age-matched controls. In comparison to the controls, peak exercise oxygen consumption (VO$_2$) was severely reduced in the patients with DHF and to a similar degree as those with SHF. Submaximal exercise capacity, as measured by the ventilatory anaerobic threshold, was similarly reduced in DHF vs. SHF patients. This was accompanied by reduced health-related quality of life.

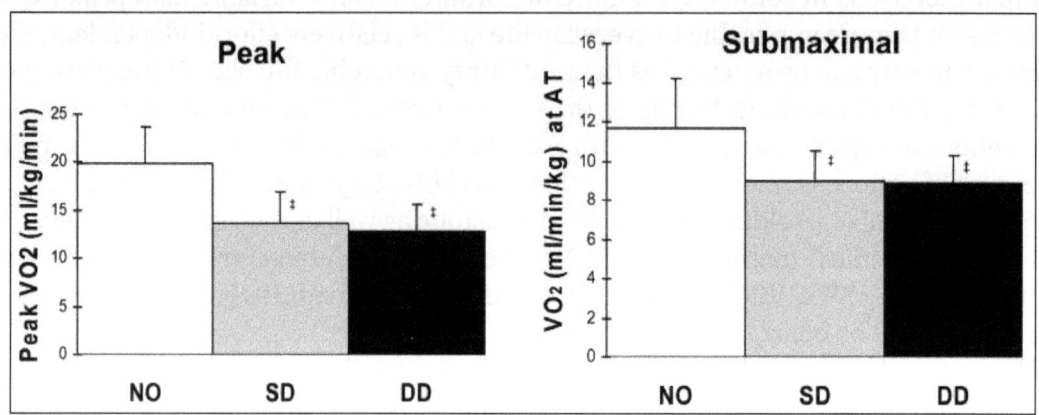

Exercise oxygen consumption (VO$_2$) during peak exhaustive exercise (left panel) and during submaximal exercise at the ventilatory anaerobic threshold (right panel) in age matched normal subjects (NO), elderly patients with heart failure due to systolic dysfunction (SD), and elderly patients with heart failure with normal systolic function, presumed diastolic dysfunction (DD). Exercise capacity is severely reduced in patients with diastolic heart failure compared to normals (p<0.001) and to a similar degree as in those with systolic heart failure. Overall, peak exercise VO$_2$ was 33% lower in the women compared to the men.

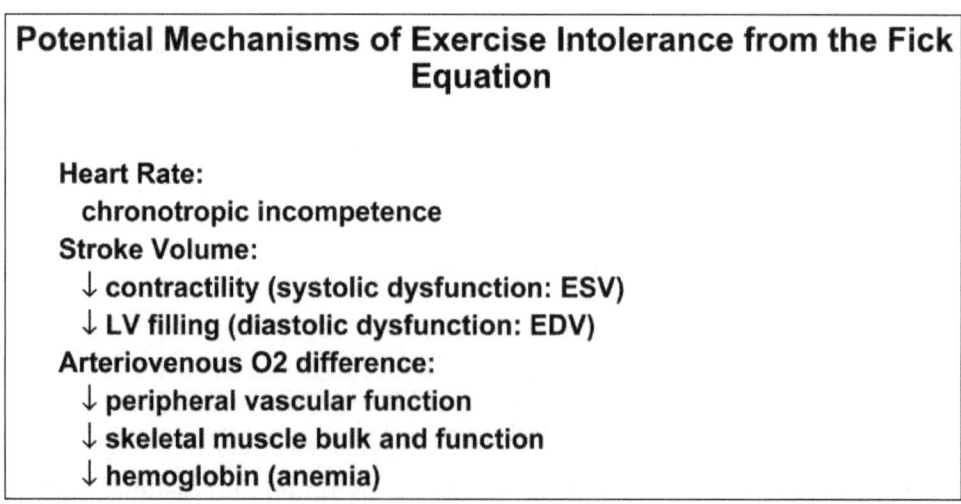

Potential mechanisms of exercise intolerance from the factors of the Fick Equation.

By the Fick equation, peak VO$_2$ during exercise is the product of cardiac output and arteriovenous oxygen (A-VO$_2$) difference, indicating that exercise intolerance will be related to one or both of these factors and to the variables that influence them. Measurement of peak exercise VO$_2$ and at least one of these other 2 factors (cardiac output or arteriovenous oxygen difference) allows one to calculate the remaining unknown factor and begin to isolate specific factors that contribute to exercise intolerance within individual patients and groups.

Central Cardiac Response to Exercise

These principles were utilized in order to examine the determinants of exercise performance in normal humans and in patients with heart failure. A series of cardiopulmonary exercise studies was performed using symptom limited upright bicycle exercise with indwelling pulmonary artery and brachial artery catheters, and simultaneous expired gas analysis and radionuclide ventriculography. Cardiac output was determined by the Fick principle for oxygen, and left ventricular end-diastolic volume and end-systolic volume were calculated from the Fick stroke volume and the radionuclide ejection fraction (LVEF).

In healthy young and middle-aged male and female volunteers during upright bicycle exercise, VO_2 increases 7.7-fold from rest to peak exercise, and this is achieved by a 3.2-fold increase in cardiac output and a 2.5-fold increase in A-V O_2 difference. The increase in cardiac output results from a 2.5-fold increase in heart rate and a 1.4-fold increase in stroke volume. Stroke volume increases during low levels of exercise via the Frank-Starling mechanism and during higher levels of exercise, stroke volume increases predominantly due to increased contractility, and may even decline slightly due to tachycardia and limited filling time.

Aging is known to be accompanied by reduced peak exercise VO_2 and this is due to an age-related declines in peak exercise cardiac output, heart rate, stroke volume and left ventricular ejection fraction. Thus, stroke volume and end diastolic volume response are important contributors to the increase in VO_2 and cardiac output during upright exercise in normal subjects and are altered by normal aging but not gender.

Invasive cardiopulmonary exercise testing was performed in 7 patients with severe but stable chronic heart failure, 6 of whom had had at least one episode of clinically and radiographically documented pulmonary edema. Patients had no significant coronary artery disease angiography, normal left ventricular ejection fraction ($\geq 50\%$), no wall motion abnormalities, and no evidence of valvular or pericardial disease. Most but not all patients had a history of hypertension and increased LV mass. Ten age-matched and gender-matched healthy volunteers served as normal controls.

The diastolic heart failure patients had marked exercise intolerance and a 48% reduction in peak oxygen consumption. In patients and normal subjects, exercise was limited primarily by leg fatigue, and dyspnea was also frequently reported. The peak respiratory exchange ratio was > 1.10 and similar in patients compared to normal subjects, suggesting good exercise effort in both groups. In both groups, arterial lactate concentration increased several fold from rest to peak exercise and during submaximal exercise at 50 watts where oxygen consumption was similar in patients and normals, lactate concentration tended to be increased in the patients compared to the normal subjects (2.2 ± 1.1 vs. 1.4 ± 0.7 mmol/liter).

At rest, there were no intergroup differences at rest in cardiac output, central A-V O_2 difference, stroke volume, or heart rate between the two groups. However, cardiac output was significantly reduced in the patients at submaximal workloads and was severely reduced by 41% at peak exercise. Central A-V O$_2$ difference was increased by approximately 10% in the patients during the submaximal exercise, partially compensating for the reduced cardiac index. However, at peak exercise, this mechanism was outstripped, and A-V O$_2$ difference was reduced by 13%. In the patients, the change in cardiac output from rest to peak exercise correlated closely with the increase in VO$_2$ during exercise (r=0.81, P<0.03).

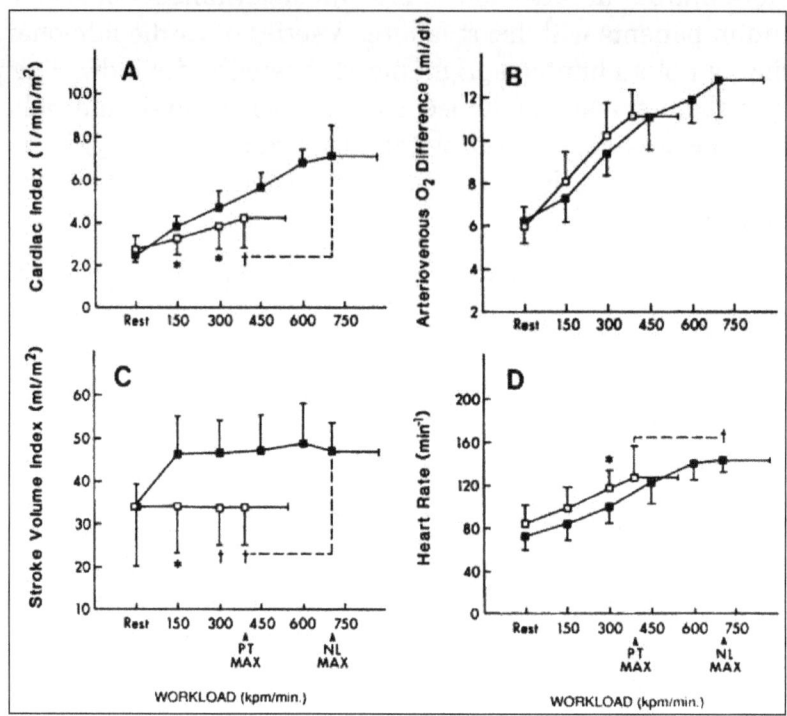

Cardiovascular function assessed by invasive cardiopulmonary exercise testing in patients with heart failure and normal systolic function (open boxes) and age-matched normals (closed boxes). The primary components of the Fick equation for oxygen consumption, cardiac output and arteriovenous oxygen difference, are shown in panels A and B, respectively. The components of cardiac output, stroke volume and heart rate, are shown in panels C and D. The X-axis is exercise workload in kpm/min; 150 kpm/min is equivalent to 25 watts.

Stroke volume was reduced in the patients during submaximal exercise and was markedly reduced (−26%) at peak exercise.Likewise, heart rate was reduced by 18% in patients compared to controls at peak exercise. The change in stroke volume correlated well with the increase in cardiac output during exercise, suggesting that in the diastolic heart failure patients, reduced stroke volume was the primary factor for reduced cardiac output and the 48% reduction in peak VO$_2$.

There are a number of possible factors that could contribute to the abnormal stroke volume response in the patients, and these are shown in Figures. The left ventricular ejection fraction and end-systolic volume index during rest and exercise were not different from the normal subjects, confirming that systolic function was within normal limits. End-diastolic volume, in contrast, was reduced markedly during exercise, resulting in a flattened curve that was similar to the abnormal stroke volume response. In the patients, the change in end-diastolic volume from rest to peak exercise correlated strongly with the change in stroke volume and in cardiac output.

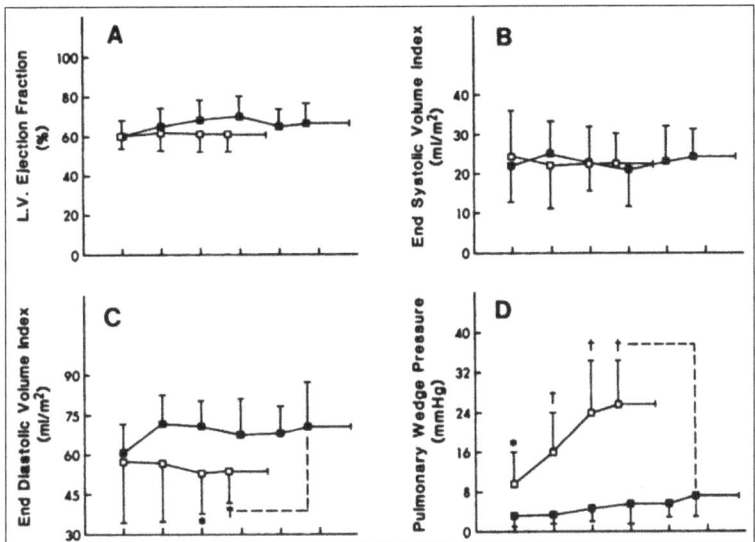

The components of the LV stroke volume response during exercise, LV ejection fraction, end-systolic volume, end-diastolic volume, and LV filling pressure, are shown in panels A–D. Not shown are systolic and mean arterial pressure, which was not different between groups.

Pulmonary wedge pressure as an estimate of LV filling pressure was mildly increased in the patients at rest and became severely increased during exercise. Notably, however, the change in pulmonary wedge pressure from rest to peak exercise did not correlate significantly with the change in stroke volume or the increase in VO_2 during exercise. The left ventricular end-diastolic pressure-volume ratio tended to be elevated in the patients at rest and during exercise became markedly increased. The upward, left-shifted left ventricular diastolic pressure-volume relationship in the DHF patients is shown in Figure and indicates that the patients did not utilize the Frank-Starling mechanism, likely primarily due to diastolic LV dysfunction. This is in contrast to patients with heart failure and reduced systolic function who have an operating pressure volume relationship that is shifted upward and to the right during exercise.

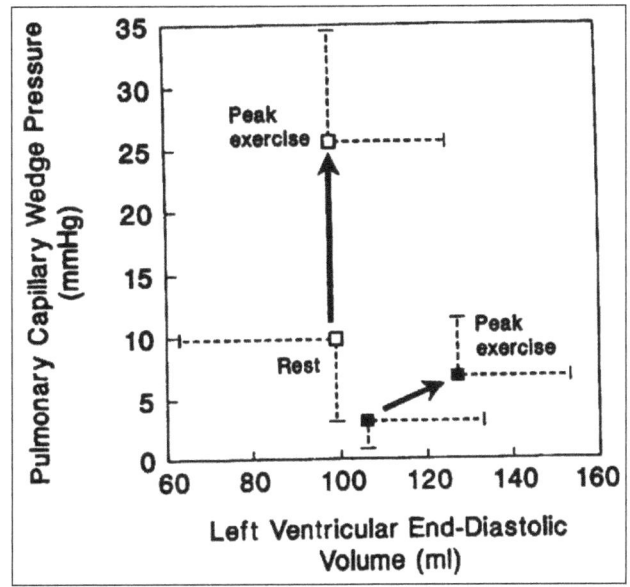

Central and Peripheral Vascular Contributions to Exercise Intolerance

Abnormal afterload and abnormal ventricular-vascular coupling may contribute to the abnormal Frank-Starling response seen in the diastolic heart failure patients. Nearly all (88%) of such patients have a history of chronic systemic hypertension. In animal models, diastolic dysfunction develops early in systemic hypertension, and LV diastolic relaxation is sensitive to increased afterload, which can impair relaxation, leading to increased LV filling pressures, decreased stroke volume, and could lead to symptoms of dyspnea and congestion.

In animal models and humans, chronic systolic hypertension accelerates and magnifies the age-related increase in fibrotic thickening of the aortic wall and resultant increase in aortic stiffness, which is a major determinant of LV afterload and ventricular-vascular coupling. To determine whether abnormally decreased aortic distensibility contributes to the severe exercise intolerance in heart failure with normal EF researchers performed magnetic resonance imaging and maximal exercise testing with expired gas analysis in a group of elderly patients with isolated DHF, as defined above, and in young healthy subjects and age-matched healthy subjects as normal controls. The patients with DHF had severe exercise intolerance, and this was associated with increased pulse pressure and concentric hypertrophic LV remodeling. Thoracic aortic wall thickness was increased 50% and there was markedly decreased aortic distensibility. In univariate analysis, decreased aortic distensibility correlated closely with their severely decreased peak exercise oxygen consumption. In multivariate analysis, decreased aortic distensibility was the strongest independent predictor of reduced exercise capacity. These data support a potentially important role of increased aortic stiffness, due to underlying aging and amplified by chronic hypertension, in the pathophysiology of chronic heart failure symptoms

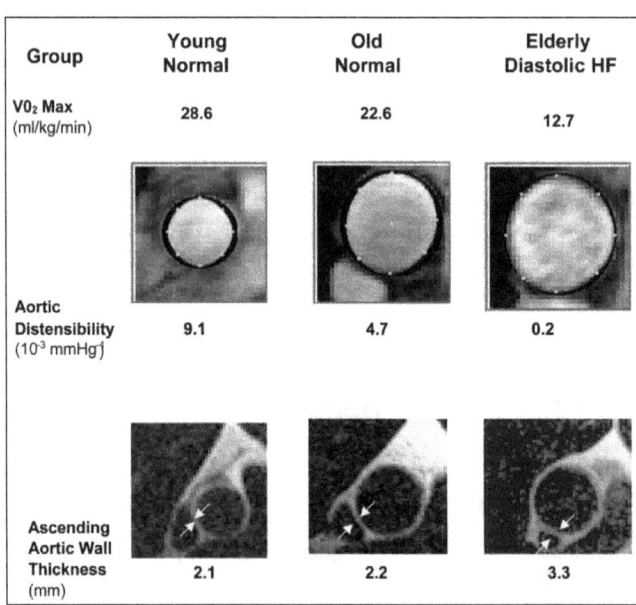

Data and images from representative subjects from healthy young, healthy elderly, and elderly patients with diastolic heart failure. Maximal exercise oxygen consumption (Vo_2max), aortic distensibility at rest, and left ventricular mass:volume ratio. Patients with diastolic heart failure have severely reduced exercise tolerance (Vo_2max) and aortic distensibility and increased aortic wall thickness.

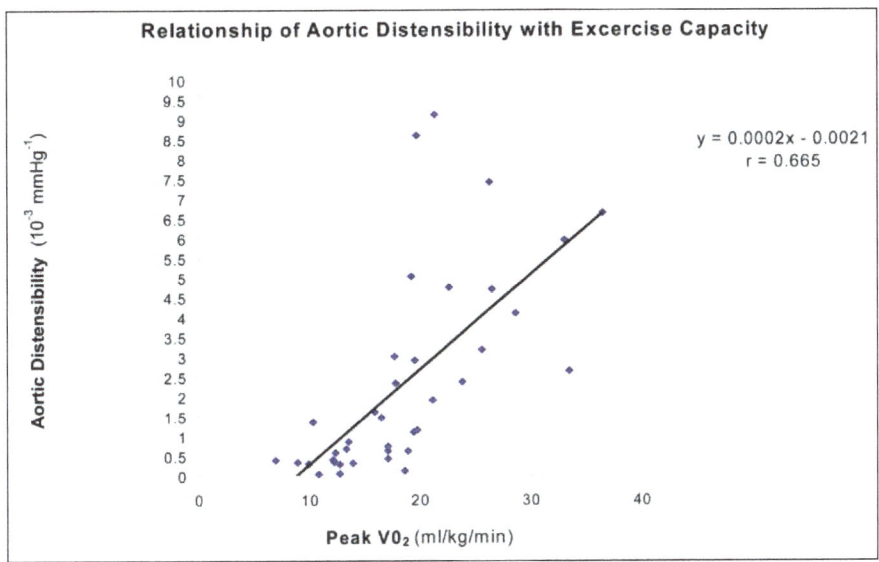

There is a close relationship between peak exercise VO_2 (horizontal axis) and proximal aortic distensibility (vertical axis) in a group of 30 subjects (10 healthy young, 10 healthy old, and 10 elderly DHF patients). Each symbol represents the data from 1 participant.

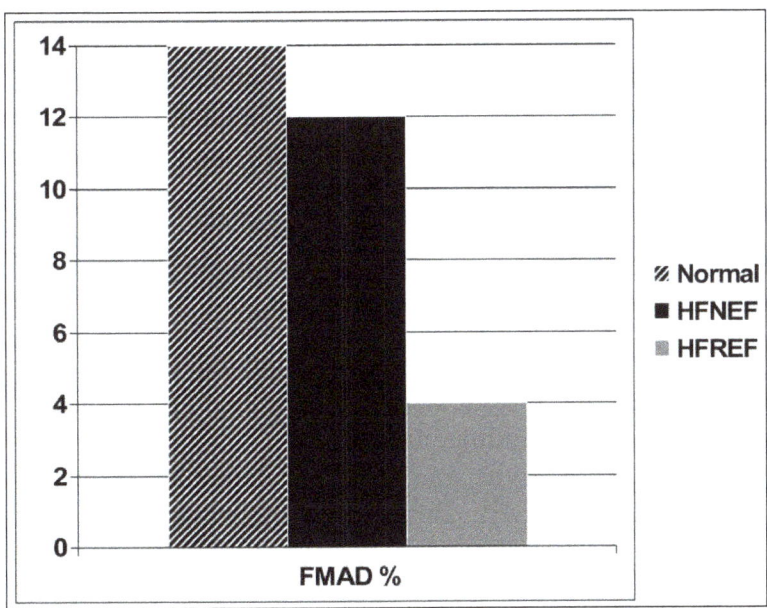

Flow mediated arterial dilation (FMAD) of the femoral artery by phase contrast magnetic resonance imaging in normal subjects, elderly patients with heart failure and normal ejection fraction (HFNEF) and patients with heart failure and reduced ejection fraction (HFREF). FMAD is severely reduced in HFREF but is relatively preserved in HFNEF compared to age matched healthy normal subjects.

Peripheral arteries must dilate early during exercise in order to accommodate and facilitate the conveyance of increased nutritive blood flow to working skeletal muscle. Multiple lines of evidence suggest that in patients with systolic heart failure, this response is impaired, and contributes to exercise intolerance, and that this is modifiable with exercise training and other interventions.

hydrochlorothiazide was compared with the angiotensin receptor antagonist losartan on the outcomes of peak exercise blood pressure, exercise time and quality of life. While both agents blunted the peak systolic blood pressure response to exercise, only losartan, but not hydrochlorothiazide, improved exercise time and quality of life.

The addition of low dose spironolactone (12.5–50 mg daily) to standard therapy has been shown to improve exercise tolerance in patients with severe SHF. Aldosterone antagonism has numerous potential benefits in patients with DHF, including LV remodeling, reversal of myocardial fibrosis, and improved LV diastolic function and vascular function. However few data are presently available regarding aldosterone antagonism in DHF. In one small study, low dose spironolactone was well tolerated and appeared to improve exercise capacity and quality of life in older women with isolated DHF. In another, spironolactone improved measures of myocardial function in hypertensive patients with diastolic heart failure.

Glucose cross-links increase with aging and diabetes, and cause increased vascular and myocardial stiffness. Alagebrium, a novel cross-link breaker, improved vascular and LV stiffness in dogs. In a small, open label, 4-month trial of this agent in elderly patients, LV mass, quality of life, and tissue Doppler diastolic function indexes improved, but there were no significant improvements in exercise capacity or aortic distensibility, the primary outcomes of the trial. A variety of other agents and strategies are currently being evaluated or under consideration for this syndrome, including a selective endothelin antagonist.

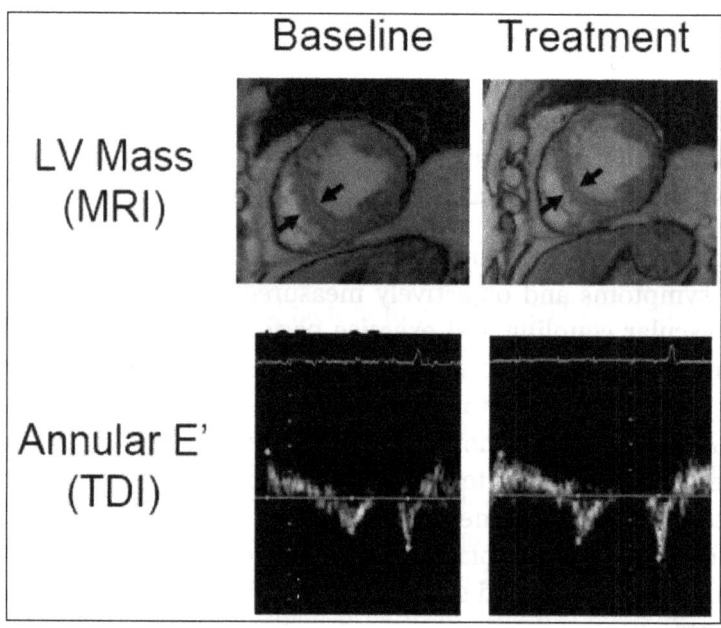

Effect of alegebrium on left ventricular mass (top panel) and tissue Doppler early diastolic velocity at the mitral annulus in older patients with diastolic heart failure.

The substantial chronotropic incompetence seen in DHF patients and its correlation with reduced exercise capacity described above provides a rationale for electronic pacing interventions to improve exercise capacity. Indeed, one modest sized single-center study used such a strategy in selected patients with hypertensive left ventricular hypertrophy with supranormal systolic ejection and distal cavity obliteration who had debilitating exertional fatigue and dyspnea and demonstrated substantially improved exercise performance. These data merit confirmation in larger, multicenter randomized controlled trials.

Thus, a variety of pharmacological and other interventions in small studies have shown improvements in exercise tolerance with verapamil, enalapril, angiotensin receceptor antagonism, and aldosterone antagonism. It should be remembered that in patients with systolic heart failure, some types of pharmacological interventions that improve exercise tolerance have had paradoxical effects on long-term survival. Because of this, VE/VCO_2 slope during exercise, which is a powerful predictor of survival independent of VO_2, should be included in future intervention trials of exercise tolerance.

Aerobic exercise training has the potential to improve a variety of key abnormalities in patients with heart failure and normal ejection fraction, including LV diastolic compliance, aortic distensibility, blood pressure, and skeletal muscle function. Indeed, in systolic heart failure, aerobic exercise training has been shown to improve exercise tolerance, likely via favorable effects on multiple factors. A recent report indicates that LV diastolic compliance is preserved in older masters athletes compared to their age matched and young counterparts, suggesting that exercise training may be beneficial in diastolic heart failure as well. A preliminary report indicates that exercise training improves exercise tolerance and quality of life in older patients with heart failure and normal ejection fraction. A recent report from a clinical exercise rehabilitation program suggests that exercise training may also benefit patients with DHF. Although the role of exercise training in the clinical management of this syndrome remains to be defined, as is the accepted practice in systolic heart failure, it would seem prudent to recommend regular, moderate physical activity as tolerated. The effect of exercise training on survival in systolic heart failure patients is being examined in a large, NIH-sponsored, multicenter, randomized, controlled trial (HF-ACTION). Presently, there is no trial examining mortality and exercise training in patients with heart failure and normal ejection fraction.

Lactate Threshold

Lactate inflection point (LIP), is the exercise intensity at which the blood concentration of lactate and/or lactic acid begins to exponentially increase. It is often expressed as 85% of maximum heart rate or 75% of maximum oxygen intake. When exercising at or below the LT, any lactate produced by the muscles is removed by the body without it building up.

The onset of blood lactate accumulation (OBLA) is often confused with the lactate threshold. With a higher exercise intensity the lactate production exceeds at a rate which it cannot be broken down, the blood lactate concentration will show an increase equal to 4.0mM; it then accumulates at the muscle and then moves to the bloodstream.

Regular endurance exercise leads to adaptations in skeletal muscle which prevent lactate levels from rising. This is mediated via activation of PGC-1α which alters the isoenzyme composition of the LDH complex and decreases the activity of the lactate generating enzyme LDHA, while increasing the activity of the lactate metabolizing enzyme LDHB.

- Charting of progress of an individual's personal journey must be judged against previous achievements and not against any form of national benchmarks.

In 1993, Dr. Margaret Whitehead proposed the concept of Physical literacy at the International Association of Physical Education and Sport for Girls and Women Congress in Melbourne, Australia. From this research, the concept and definition of physical literacy was developed. In addition, the implications of physical literacy being the goal of all structures were drawn up. Since 1993 to the present day, much has been done to advance physical literacy. Research has been conducted on Physical Literacy and presented at conferences around the world. In addition, the book Physical Literacy: throughout the life course was written and numerous conferences and workshops have been delivered, to train educators, parents, health practitioners, early childhood educators, coaches, and more.

The concept of physical literacy has been developed over many years. It is seen, by a growing number of people, as the goal of the school subject, physical education. However, whilst this is extremely relevant, it is important to recognise that physical literacy is not restricted to the school years – it is relevant throughout the lifecourse. In this respect, six phases of physical literacy have been identified: infancy, childhood, adolescence, young adulthood, adulthood and older adulthood.

Over the past few years there has been considerable interest, worldwide, in the concept of physical literacy. In Great Britain, a number of local authorities have adopted it as an overall guiding principle for their work in school-based physical education. In countries such as Northern Ireland and Canada, physical literacy has been the focus for considerable rethinking in respect of children's physical development and has consequently been the inspiration behind the development of new programmes.

However, there have been a number of interpretations of the concept that have moved away from the central tenets of physical literacy. For example, in some instances physical literacy has been the name given to a programme of fundamental movement skills, implying that the concept is solely about the acquisition of physical competence. Other interpretations have focused on knowledge and understanding, particularly in the games context. Both these scenarios include elements of physical literacy, but do not represent the whole story.

Attributes

A physically literate individual will display the following attributes:

- Physical literacy can be described as a disposition characterised by the motivation to capitalise on innate movement potential to make a significant contribution to the quality of life.

- All human beings exhibit this potential. However, its specific expression will depend on individuals' endowment in respect of all capabilities, significantly their movement potential, and will be particular to the culture in which they live.

- Individuals who are physically literate will move with poise, economy and confidence in a wide variety of physically challenging situations.

- Physically literate individuals will be perceptive in 'reading' all aspects of the physical environment, anticipating movement needs or possibilities and responding appropriately to these with intelligence and imagination.

- These individuals will have a well-established sense of self as embodied in the world. This, together with an articulate interaction with the environment, will engender positive self-esteem and self-confidence.

- Sensitivity to and awareness of embodied capability will lead to fluent self-expression through non-verbal communication and to perceptive and empathetic interaction with others.

- In addition, physically literate individuals will have the ability to identify and articulate the essential qualities that influence the effectiveness of their own movement performance, and will have an understanding of the principles of embodied health with respect to basic aspects such as exercise, sleep and nutrition.

Physical Literacy Worldwide

One element of Physical literacy is the mastering of basic human movements, fundamental movement skills and fundamental sport skills that permit a child to read their environment and make appropriate decisions, allowing them to move confidently and with control in a wide range of physical activity situations. Physical literacy is the foundation of long-term participation and performance to the best of one's ability. Physical Literacy is the cornerstone of both participation and excellence in physical activity and sport. Ideally, physical literacy is developed prior to the adolescent growth spurt.

Fundamental Movement Skills and Fundamental Sport Skills

Fundamental movement skills play a significant role in a child's physical development. When a child is confident and competent in these skills, children can develop sport-specific and complex movement skills as well as enjoy a long life of physical activity. To become physically literate children need to master the 13 fundamental movement skills:

The Locomotor and Body Skills:

- Walking

- Running

- Balance

- Skating/Skiing

- Jumping

- Swimming

- Cycling

- Skipping

The Sending Skills:

- Throwing

Examples of vigorous physical activity include jogging and running (either outdoors or on a treadmill), playing tennis, swimming laps, playing basketball or soccer, or doing calisthenics like push-ups and jumping jack. Any of these activities can be done with varying levels of effort. The key for vigorous-intensity physical activity is that the activity must be performed with intense effort. You will definitely know you are exercising.

Vigorous intensity physical activity may be performed less frequently than moderate-intensity physical activity, as it is more demanding on the body.

References

- Mcpartland, darren; pree, adrian; malpeli, robert; telford, amanda (2010). Nelson physical education studies for wa. Australia: nelson. Isbn 9780170182027

- Exercise-is-medicine-the-importance-of-exercise-as-preventative-medicine-for-a-disease-free-lifestyl, fitness-medicine: intechopen.com, Retrieved 18 April, 2019

- Faude, o; kindermann, w; meyer, t (2009). "lactate threshold concepts; how valid are they?". Sports medicine. 39 (6): 469–490. Doi:10.2165/00007256-200939060-00003

- Whitehead, m (2010). Physical literacy throughout the lifecourse. London and new york: routledge. Pp. 12–14. Isbn 978-0-415-48743-6

- What are fundamental movement skills? | coaching association of canada". Www.coach.ca. Retrieved 2019-02-03

- Met-the-standard-metabolic-equivalent: verywellfit.com, Retrieved 27 May, 2019

- Shaw i, shaw bs (2014). "resistance training and the prevention of sports injuries". In hopkins g (ed.). Sports injuries: prevention, management and risk factors. Hauppauge, ny: nova science publishers. Isbn 9781634633055

Permissions

Index